Sickle Cell Disease

Edited by Osaro Erhabor

Published in London, United Kingdom

Sickle Cell Disease
http://dx.doi.org/10.5772/intechopen.98091
Edited by Osaro Erhabor

Contributors
Samit Ghosh, Francoise Bernaudin, Suzanne Verlhac, Mohammed Lafi Al-Otaibi, Osaro Erhabor, Teddy Charles Adias, Tosan Erhabor, Osaro Mgbere, Sadiya Usman, S., Egenti B.N, David-Zacharie Issom, Mara Rissatto-Lago

First published in London, United Kingdom, 2022 by IntechOpen
IntechOpen is the global imprint of INTECHOPEN LIMITED, registered in England and Wales, registration number: 11086078, 5 Princes Gate Court, London, SW7 2QJ, United Kingdom

British Library Cataloguing-in-Publication Data
A catalogue record for this book is available from the British Library

Additional hard and PDF copies can be obtained from orders@intechopen.com

Sickle Cell Disease
Edited by Osaro Erhabor
p. cm.
Print ISBN 978-1-80355-594-2
Online ISBN 978-1-80355-595-9
eBook (PDF) ISBN 978-1-80355-596-6

Meet the editor

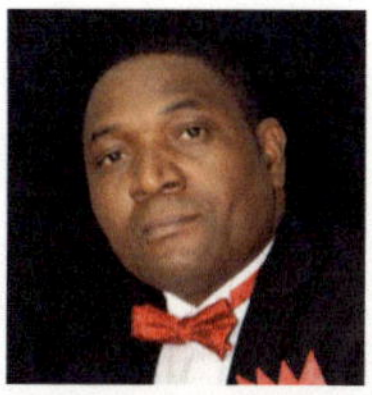

Professor Erhabor Osaro is a Chartered Scientist and Fellow of the Institute of Biomedical Science (FIBMS), British Blood Transfusion Society (BBTS), Medical Laboratory Science Council (FMLSCN), and West African Postgraduate College of Medical Laboratory Science (FWAPCMLS). He holds a Ph.D. in Immunohematology from the Rivers State University of Science and Technology, Nigeria. He completed specialist training in Blood Transfusion and Laboratory Total Quality Management at the University of Greenwich, UK. He holds a Specialist Certificate in Transfusion Science Practice (SCTSP) from the British Blood Transfusion Society (BBTS). He is an alumnus of Francis Tuttle College of Technology, Oklahoma, USA. His teaching experience spans both the African continent and the United Kingdom. Dr. Osaro is the chairman of the Blood Transfusion Faculty of the West African Postgraduate College of Medical Laboratory Science. He is a council member and chairman of the Equality and Diversity Working Group of the BBTS. He is a recipient of several academic and professional awards including the Margaret Kenwright Scientist award. He is a registration and specialist portfolio verifier/examiner for the Institute of Biomedical Science of London. He has authored several scientific books and chapters and more than 160 articles on infectious diseases, occupational health, immunohematology, and transfusion medicine. Dr. Osaro is also an editorial board member and reviewer for several international scientific journals.

Contents

Preface

Sickle cell anemia is a preventable yet prevalent inherited blood disorder. It arises due to the inheritance of two abnormal sickle cell genes (SS), one from each parent. The disease is a common cause of mortality and morbidity, particularly in low-income developing countries. The vaso-occlusive crisis is the most common presentation and the leading cause of death in patients with the disease. Its pathophysiology involves the obstruction of blood flow to vital organs by the sickled red cells resulting in ischemia, necrosis, and pain. This book presents evidence-based best practices in the diagnosis and clinical, psychosocial, and pharmacological management of sickle cell disease patients. It contains cutting-edge and evidence-based information and is highly recommended for all healthcare professionals responsible for managing patients with sickle cell disease. There is no doubt that this book will improve the quality of care offered to patients across the globe.

Osaro Erhabor
Professor,
Usmanu Danfodiyo University,
Sokoto, Nigeria

Section 1

Complications and Management of Sickle Cell Disease

Chapter 1

A Vascular Necrosis of Femoral Head in Sickle Cell Anemia

Mohammed Lafi Al-Otaibi

Abstract

Sickle cell disease is a well-known disease with evolving changes in medical as well as surgical management. Recent developments in medical management and the well-adjusted screening protocols for the disease complications toward its anticipation and prevention and all these recent changes have led to more work toward understanding and managing disease orthopedics complications. Many researchers considered the major ones affecting patients' daily living activity, with the improvement in patients living expectancy. Thanks to the evidence-based medical management and the development of new agents such as L-Glutamate that are recently implemented and help space the vaso-occlusive crises. This phenomenon plays the cornerstone effects on the disease pathology and leads to its harmful effects on many systems, including the muscles and bones. The infarct does occur almost everywhere through the muscle-skeletal system, with predilected site happening to be the hip joints. A vascular necrosis of the femoral head does occur in other conditions, and dealing with the one happening in sickle cell anemia must take into account all issues concerning this disease. There is growing evidence that surgical intervention with the total hip is best when there is a loss of congruency of the femoral head with head subchondral collapse and not in pure infarct with femoral head maintaining its sphere shape.

Keywords: bone infarct, hip pain, hip replacement, hip score, secondary arthritis, sickle cell anemia, osteonecrosis

1. Introduction

The presence of a heterozygous glutamic acid to valine substitution on chromosome 11 in the β-globin gene is known as sickle cell trait, which is found in around 300 million individuals across the globe [1]. In comparison to the homozygous genotype (HbSS) in individuals who have sickle cell disease, individuals with sickle cell trait possess heterozygous genotype (HbAS).

Over the years, few bone complications have been reported in sickle cell trait that is back in the 1970s era [2]. It is pretty uncommon that people with sickle cell trait suffer from a vascular necrosis (AVN) of bone and femoral head as the most common destruction site [3].

Multifactorial etiology is investigated for nontraumatic a vascular necrosis of the femoral head. In the majority of the cases (30–70%), both the hips are affected by the lesion [4]. The cause of AVN of the head of the femur is yet unknown. However, several risk factors have been linked to the development of this disease.

Sickle cell anemia, alcohol consumption/abuse, hemoglobinopathies, myeloproliferative disorders, chemotherapy, pregnancy, genetic susceptibility are chronic steroid usage, smoking, coagulopathies, leukemia, ionizing irradiation, and HIV infection are considered as the main risk factors [4]. The fundamental pathophysiologic cause of osteonecrosis in sickle cell disease is the obstruction of micro vessels, resulting in ischemia and oxygen and nutrition deprivation of the afflicted bone [5].

Sickle cell disease is the most common cause of osteonecrosis in children, with a prevalence incidence of 3% before 15 years. Sickle cell trait is thought to be primarily protective, particularly in the case of malaria. Despite this therapeutic benefit, afflicted carriers might have various problems and clinical sequelae, including exercise-related injury, venous thromboembolism, and renal difficulties [1, 6].

The possibility of AVN of the femoral head in sickle cell trait was reported by Perumal and Corbett [7]; however, there is a need for additional research. This index case describes and raises awareness of a vascular necrosis of the femoral head and its relationship to sickle cell trait.

The autosomal recessive genetic disorder sickle cell disease is marked by abnormal sickle hemoglobin synthesis and reduced pliability of red blood cells. It causes blood arteries to clog, resulting in ischemia and infarction of the afflicted tissue [8]. Despite being indigenous to tropical Africa and the Middle East, it has become a worldwide disease due to population movement [9].

One of the most prevalent sickle cell disease clinical signs is bone involvement, which can vary from an acute severe vaso-occlusive crisis to a persistent impairment such as a vascular necrosis. Pathological fractures, septic arthritis, osteonecrosis, and osteomyelitis are orthopedic consequences of sickle cell disease [10].

The most common location for a vascular necrosis in sickle cell disease is the femoral head, followed by the shoulder, knee, and other minor joints [11]. A vascular necrosis of the femoral head causes hip osteoarthritis and reduces its functional capability. To avoid morbidity and mortality associated with late diagnosis, osteonecrosis must be diagnosed early and treated promptly. The majority of orthopedic surgeons advocate complete hip replacement to increase functional capacity [12].

In sickle cell disease patients, aberrant metaphyseal femoral morphology with thin cortices and trabeculae, low bone density, and medullary hyperplasia are only a few skeletal abnormalities that affect the hip joint. The femoral canal can also be obliterated by irregular bone sclerotic regions, resulting in hip joint congruency loss. Thinned femoral cortical lining inside the outer cortex might sometimes seem like a femur inside a femur [13].

The disturbance in the proximal femur's blood supply causes a vascular necrosis of the femoral head, known as osteonecrosis. Each year, between 10,000 and 20,000 new cases are recorded in the United States alone [14]. It can be caused by a multitude of factors, both traumatic and nontraumatic. Fractures, dislocations, chronic steroid usage, prolonged alcohol use, coagulopathy, and congenital reasons are only a few of the causes.

A vascular necrosis of the femoral head is a devastating illness requiring healthcare providers to look for its symptoms. This exercise will provide you with a summary of the etiology and treatment options, as well as some clinical pearls.

The lateral and medial circumflex branches of the profunda femoris, which is a branch of the femoral artery, give the bulk of the blood flow to the head of the femur. It is known that the profunda femoris is the deep penetrating branch present in the upper thigh region. A ring around the femur's neck is created by joining medial and lateral circumflex femoral arteries. This is the place from which many tiny arteries branch for perfusing the femoral head.

The foveal artery, also known as the ligamentum teres artery, is another direct route of blood flow. The femur head is linked to the acetabulum through the ligamentum teres. The foveal artery flows through the ligament, but its contribution is only noticeable in children [15].

Two significant anastomoses provide collateral blood flow for supporting femoral; although, the flow is limited;

- Cruciate anastomosis—it maintains flow between medial circumflex femoral and inferior gluteal artery.

- trochanteric anastomosis—it maintains flow between medial/lateral circumflex femoral and superior gluteal artery.

The internal iliac artery, also known as the hypogastric artery, is the major artery of the pelvis and nourishes a portion of the buttock and posterior thigh [15]. The common iliac artery is derived from the aorta, and the internal iliac artery is derived from it.

The socket of the hip, the acetabulum, is the place where the femoral head is connected. The acetabular branch of the obturator artery provides blood supply to the acetabulum, along with the deep branches of the superior gluteal artery and pubic branches of the obturator artery. Disruption of the blood flow to the head of the femur might produce ischemia and necrosis due to restricted collateral circulation. The osteocytes will die, the articular surface will crumble, and degenerative arthritis will develop if the blood supply is not restored quickly [16].

2. Etiology

The etiology of AVN of the femur head is not well established. But several conditions have been regarded as risk factors for its development.

The dislocation and fracture involving femoral neck fracture and the acetabulum are among the most common traumatic causes. A vascular necrosis can result during sorts due to damage of the blood supply to the head of the femur, which is easily disturbed in some traumas associated with sport activities. In total, 15–50% of femur neck fractures and 10–25% of hip dislocations are caused by osteonecrosis [17].

Most nontraumatic etiologies are represented through increased alcohol use and chronic use of steroids, accounting for >80% of the cases. After trauma, the second most common cause of osteonecrosis is steroid-associated osteonecrosis. The actual pathogenesis is unknown and most likely complex despite indications of an association between steroids and osteonecrosis. Fat emboli, fat cell hypertrophy leading to increased endothelial dysfunction, bone marrow stem cell pool abnormalities, intraosseous pressure, and hyperlipidemia are all possible contributors to ischemia and necrosis [18].

There is a lack of understanding about alcohol-induced osteonecrosis. However, proliferation, bone marrow fat cell hypertrophy, blood vessel occlusion, subsequent lack of perfusion, changes in serum lipid levels, and increased intraosseous pressure are known to cause osteonecrosis [19].

Osteonecrosis is frequently triggered by sickle cell disease. Ischemia and bone infarction result from the malformed inflexible red blood cells, with the femoral head being the most prevalent location of osteonecrosis in these patients [20]. Autoimmune and chronic inflammatory illnesses, such as systemic lupus erythematosus, have long been linked to femoral head osteonecrosis. Long-term steroid therapy is frequently related to developing the illness in these people, while there have been instances among steroid naïve.

Perthes, which affects the pediatric population due to idiopathic a vascular necrosis of the femoral head. There is an increased risk of osteoarthritis and losing range of motion due to lack of blood supply resulting in necrosis of the femoral head leading to deformity. The progression of disease takes place in four steps as follows [21];

- Necrosis—it is when necrosis begins due to disruption of blood supply.
- Fragmentation—resorption of necrotic bone takes place that is replaced with woven bone, with increased susceptibility of either collapsing or breaking.
- Re-ossification—development of stronger bone.
- Bone remodeling—completion of bone regrowth and finalized shape, considering the damage caused during the second phase of fragmentation.

The development of femoral head osteonecrosis has also been linked to vascular disease caused by diabetes and direct injury by cytotoxic chemicals [22].

3. Epidemiology

A vascular necrosis of the femoral head is expected to develop at a rate of 20,000–30,000 new cases each year in the United States, accounting for 10% of the approximately 250,000 total hip arthroplasties performed each year [23]. This number is comparable to the 0.01% incidence observed in German-speaking nations and the 1.9 per 100,000 incidences reported in Japan.

There is no link between race and sickness, except in cases of sickle cell disease, which is more common among people of African heritage. Overall, men are more likely than women to have this illness, with studies predicting ratios ranging from 3 to 5 to 1 [24]. The average age of the patients at the time of therapy is between 33 and 38 years old [14].

4. Pathophysiology

The actual pathophysiologic processes behind a vascular necrosis of the femoral head are not always evident, and the condition is commonly thought to be complex [4]. The consequence is the death of osteocytes and bone marrow due to inadequate blood supply to the subchondral bone of the proximal femur, regardless of the causative event [17]. If not treated adequately in the early stages, this cell loss will collapse the femoral head and subsequent osteoarthritis. It is also clear in literature that the AVN is inevitable end result in some conditions.

5. History of the disease

Early on in the illness phase, patients may be asymptomatic. However, when they become symptomatic, the most common complaint is hip discomfort that might extend to the groin and thigh. Activities such as climbing stairs and walking worsen the discomfort, which is relieved by relaxation. Even when there is no movement, the pain will often persist [4]. Restricted range of motion, soreness on palpation, and discomfort during abduction and internal rotation of the hip area are some physical exam findings suggestive of femoral head osteonecrosis.

Total hip replacement is one of the most satisfying procedures and has been dubbed the "century surgery" due to its nearly 50-year track record of success [25]. Total hip replacement became popular in the 1960s to restore hip function and, as a result, everyday activities. Since then, surgical technique and surgeon training advancements have led to today's condition of high-quality prosthetic implants, well-proven surgical indications and contraindications, and evidence-based pre- and postoperative treatment.

On average, 85–95% of hip replacement patients survive [26]. Total hip replacement for sickle anemia is a complicated treatment with medical, intraoperative, and postoperative problems. The success necessary to medically optimize patients and improvements in surgical procedures and prosthetic implant manufacturing has yielded equivalent outcomes for sickle cell anemia patients.

Adherence to proper perioperative measures such as hydration, body temperature management, oxygenation, and a hemoglobin level of over 10 mg/dl contributes favorably to the outcome and is relatively simple to implement. Intraoperative complications such as soft tissue contractures, bone fractures, and perforations are challenging to manage and are a primary cause of poor results [27].

There is a need for further improvement for a hip replacement among the affected individuals, considering the impact of bony involvement such as scoliosis or soft tissue conditions. One such condition is Periarticular Contracture on hip replacement such as degenerative hip and spine for sickle cell anemia elderly patients.

6. Evaluating sickle cell disease

Early detection can have a significant impact on the result. The clinical presentation is combined with adequate imaging to make a diagnosis. X-rays, radionuclide bone scanning, and magnetic resonance imaging (MRI) are all examples of imaging. Imaging in the context of a patient's symptoms can aid in determining the best course of treatment.

Usually, the plain-film radiography is performed in two planes, using both frog-leg lateral and anterior–posterior films. Subchondral radiolucency, often known as the "crescent sign," is a pathognomonic indication of subchondral collapse. The "donut sign," which is a ring of enhanced uptake around a chilly core, might appear when Technetium-99 m is absorbed. At the demarcation, where reactive bone meets dead bone, this indication signifies increased bone turnover [23].

The gold standard for diagnosing osteonecrosis is an MRI. X-rays and radionuclide scans can also help diagnose, but none is as sensitive or accurate as MRI to detect radiographic evidence early in disease development. When determining a patient's prognosis and devising a treatment plan, MRI can identify bone marrow alterations, the size/location of the necrotic region, the influence on acetabular cartilage, the depth of collapse, and so on [4].

The amount of necrosis can be classified if appropriate imaging has been obtained. While there are other staging systems available, the Steinberg staging system is the most often utilized. It specifies the seven stages illustrated in **Table 1**.

In patients with suspected osteonecrosis, a laboratory workup should be performed to help rule out alternative causes of hip pain and check for concomitant conditions. The lipid panel, C-reactive protein (CRP), anti-nuclear antibody (ANA), hemoglobin electrophoresis, a complete blood count (CBC), erythrocyte sedimentation rate (ESR), rheumatoid factor (RF), and anti-cyclic citrullinated peptide (anti-CCP) are some of the tests that may be used in a workup.

Elevated ANA and RF are nonspecific indicators of active autoimmune disease. Inflammatory processes raise both ESR and CRP. However, they are nonspecific. Rheumatoid arthritis is associated with elevated anti-CCP antibodies, whereas sickle cell disease is associated with HbS and a low quantity of HbF on hemoglobin electrophoresis [28].

A CBC with indications of normocytic or microcytic anemia and a high reticulocyte count is also constant with a sickle cell disease diagnosis. Sickle cell disease and rheumatoid arthritis are two disorders that can lead to femoral head osteonecrosis and produce hip discomfort even if there is no osteonecrosis.

A biopsy is rarely required because the diagnosis can frequently be determined precisely based on imaging and clinical presentation. If a biopsy is taken, the typical histological results will be trabecular necrosis (more than 50% empty osteocytic

Stage	Features
0	Normal radiograph, bone scan, and MRI
I	Normal radiograph, abnormal bone scan, and or magnetic resonance imaging IA Mild (involves less than 15% of the femoral head). IB Moderate (involves 15–30% of the femoral head) IC Severe (affects over 30% of the femoral head)
II	Cystic and sclerotic change of the femoral head IIA Mild (involves less than 15% of the femoral head) IIB Moderate (affects 15–30% of the femoral head) IIC Severe (affects more than 30% of the femoral head)
III	Subchondral collapse (crescent sign) without flattening of the femoral head IIIA Mild (involves under 15% of the femoral head) IIIB Moderate (affects 15–30% of the femoral head) IIIC Severe (affects over 30% of the femoral head)
IV	Flattening of the femoral head/femoral head collapse IVA Mild (involves under 15% of the femoral head) IVB Moderate (involves 15–30% of the femoral head) IVC Severe (affects more significant than 30% of the femoral head)
V	Joint space narrowing and acetabular changes VA Mild VB Moderate VC Severe
VI	Advanced degenerative joint disease

Table 1.
Steinberg staging system [23].

lacunae) and necrotic hematopoietic marrow, with no signs of inflammation, tumor cells, or sepsis [29]. Similarly, angiography tests are rarely regularly conducted, despite their excellent vasculature imaging, and may aid in disease pathology research [28, 30].

7. Disease management

A vascular necrosis of the femoral head can be treated in different ways, such as they can be treated through conservative to invasive methods. The particular therapy used is determined on the basis of the patient's condition individually along with a variety of circumstances for optimal results. All considered are the patient's age, location and extent of necrosis, comorbidities, amount of pain/discomfort, and whether the articular surface has collapsed. Treatments, which include both operational and non-operative approaches, are best applied during the pre-collapse period. Femoral head necrosis, if left untreated, can develop subchondral fractures in as little as 2–3 years [31].

Treatment options should be depending on the severity of the lesions, but primarily on whether or not they have collapsed. In asymptomatic and symptomatic small to medium-sized pre-collapse lesions, non-operative therapies or core decompression can be beneficial. Bone grafts (non-vascularized or vascularized) or osteotomies can be used to treat medium-to-large lesions. Arthroplasty is recommended if there is femoral collapse or acetabular involvement.

The term "conservative management" refers to a group of non-operative therapies. Physical therapy, reduced weight-bearing, alcohol abstinence, steroid discontinuance, pain management medication, and focused pharmacologic treatment are only a few examples. Because the time it takes for a vascular necrosis of the femoral head to develop and collapse varies widely, and data are poor, there is no consensus on conservative therapies. Despite the fact that minor asymptomatic lesions can heal independently, the majority develop and require treatment.

Off-label usage of statins, anticoagulants, vasodilators, and bisphosphonates has been attempted to revascularize the femoral head. Vasodilators, such as iloprost (PGI2), work by lowering intraosseous pressure and increasing blood flow [32]. Statins inhibit the development of stem cells into fat cells, lowering intraosseous pressure and improving perfusion [33]. Anticoagulants such as enoxaparin are used to prevent osteonecrosis from progressing due to thromboembolic events and hypercoagulability [34]. Bisphosphonates, such as alendronate, block osteoclasts' ability to reduce bone resorption [35].

There is still no significant consensus on the efficacy of any of these drugs over another, despite the availability of a multitude of pharmacologic treatment options. In general, intra-articular steroid injections are not advised. The benefits of steroid injections are generally fleeting, and their usage might exacerbate a vascular necrosis; although, they can give pain relief.

For individuals who require more intrusive therapy, there are many surgical choices. They are classified as either joint preservation techniques or joint reconstruction procedures. Bone grafts, osteotomy, core decompression, biologics, and cellular treatments are examples of joint preservation operations, whereas joint replacement is an example of reconstructive interventions.

The lateral approach was used for all surgeries. The incision was made around 8 cm down the line of the femur, 5 cm proximal to the tip of the greater trochanter longitudinal incision centered over, the greater trochanter's tip. The fascia lata was split and retracted anteriorly during the superficial dissection, exposing the gluteus medius tendon.

The gluteus medius fibers that were connected to the fascia lata were removed using sharp dissection. Deep dissection separated the gluteus medius fibers longitudinally, commencing in the center of the greater trochanter and extending the incision inferiorly via the vastus lateralis fibers to avoid harm to the superior gluteal nerve [10]. The anterior greater trochanter and its underlying gluteus minimus formed an anterior flap in the anterior gluteus medius.

To expose the anterior joint capsule, the anterior region of the vastus lateralis needed forceful dissection of the muscles from the bone or lifting specks of bone where possible. Following anterior dissection down the greater trochanter and onto the femoral neck, the gluteus minimus capsule was freed from the anterior greater trochanter, allowing for simple hip dislocation.

To avoid problems or fractures, enough exposure and attentive soft-tissue manipulation were used. In patients with a sclerotic and constricted femoral canal, extra measures were used during femoral stem preparation [10]. To avoid femoral stem perforation, sequential reaming over guidewire was performed.

The patients are likely to get routine physical therapy for total hip replacement after surgery, including patient education, pain management, range of motion, and muscle-strengthening activities. Partially weight-bearing was allowed for the first 6 weeks, followed by full weight-bearing. Ten to twenty-one days after surgery, the patients were discharged from the hospital.

The most common intervention during pre-collapse phases is core decompression, which involves the surgical removal (by drilling) of damaged tissue from the interior of the femoral head to reduce pressure and enhance perfusion. Cell treatments have been utilized as adjuvants to core decompression. They have been found to be safe, with better clinical results and a lower rate of disease progression than core decompression alone [36, 37].

However, core decompression shows good results, and it is considered a good option for symptomatic small to medium-sized pre-collapse lesions. It is not recommended in case of a collapsed femoral head.

Bone grafting is a therapy option for more extensive lesions that do not collapse prematurely. The bone graft is likely to be obtained as a vascularized bone graft from another part of the patient's body along with intact vasculature, an autograph from another part of the patient's body, or an allograft from another person via a bone bank. The vascularized bone transplant has the extra benefit of transporting a fresh blood supply, which can help with revascularization and perhaps revitalize the necrotic zone.

The removal of segments of bone to change the weight distribution of the joint to the healthy, uninvolved bone is known as osteotomy. Angular intertrochanteric or rotational trans-trochanteric operations, in which the necrotic portion of the femoral head is shifted away from weight-bearing regions, supposedly enabling healing or slowing development [38], are common examples.

If the injury is severe, the hip has collapsed, and/or there is acetabular involvement, arthroplasty (removal of the ball-and-socket joint and replacement with a prosthesis) may be necessary [23]. While there have been improvements in hardware such as low-wear surface bearings that have significantly improved the outcome of hip replacement in the setting of osteonecrosis in the last 20 years [4], the outcome of hip replacement in the setting of osteonecrosis has previously shown mixed success rates.

The patients who underwent congruous hip joint radiologically were diagnosed to have infarct area > 30% through magnetic resonance imaging. These patients are likely to have previous joint preservation treatments (core decompression); however, pain alleviation did not seem to benefit from them. The patients undergoing an incongruent hip joint with arthritic alterations are likely to use an uncemented complete hip replacement (**Figures 1–3**).

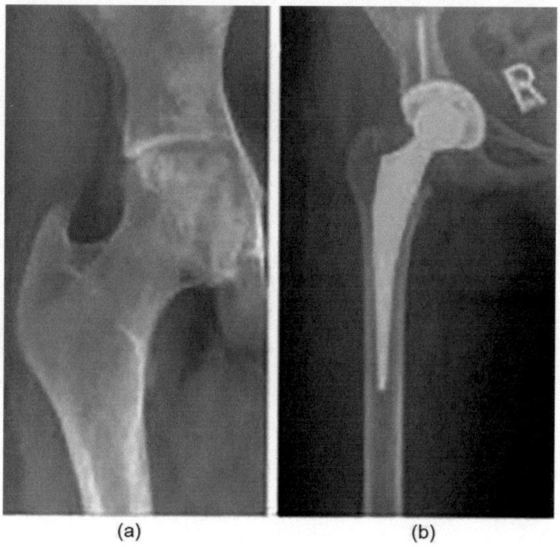

Figurc 1.
(a) Preoperative hip joint with subchondral collapse and loss of acetabular congruency; (b) postoperative hip joint with a prosthesis.

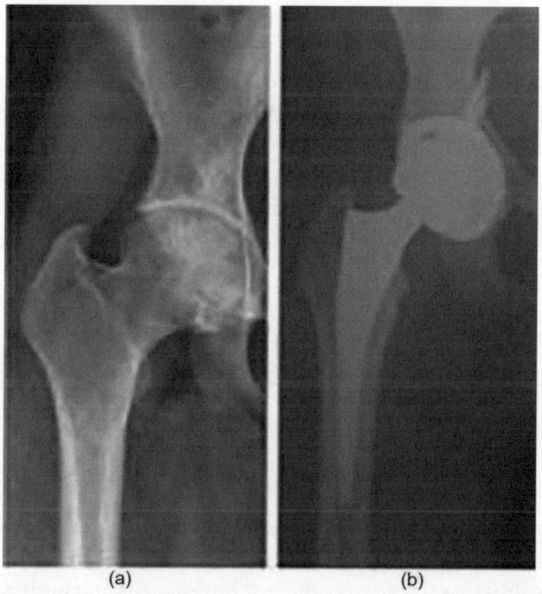

Figure 2.
(a) Preoperative hip joint with preserved acetabular congruency; (b) postoperative hip joint with a prosthesis.

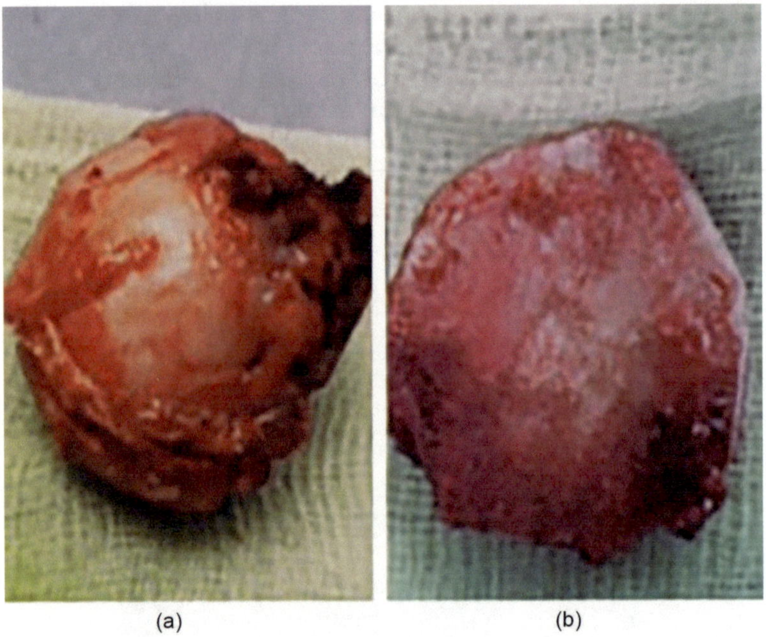

Figure 3.
Postsurgical head of the femurs; (a) Femur's round head; (b) Femur's triangular head.

8. Musculoskeletal changes

Surgical treatment, such as total hip replacement, is the last resort to address the changes occurring in the hip joint due to a vascular necrosis and secondary osteoarthritis in sickle cell anemia, even though there are less invasive procedures such as core decompression and trap door procedure that can and should be offered earlier to alter the situation.

It is important to remember that the presence of soft tissue changes such as contracture or infection, as well as skeletal findings such as the loss of the medullary canal, variation in bone quality, bone load resistance, and spine vertebral segmental collapse with a vascular necrosis, all affect the outcome of total hip replacement. Patients with just hip joint alterations are likely to have a better prognosis, but those with multiple musculoskeletal changes are expected to have a range of outcomes.

There is the proportional correlation of medullary obliteration acetabular periarticular infarct (**Figure 4a** and **b**), spine vertebral column collapse with kyphoscoliosis (**Figure 5**), and soft tissue hip and knee contractures (**Figure 6**) with the severity of preoperative symptoms, postoperative Harris Hip Scores (HHSs), and intraoperative difficulties. Other characteristics contributing to a lower hip score include severe leg length disparity, obliteration of the medullary cavities, soft tissue contractures, and poor bone quality [39].

Sickle cell disease is linked to a variety of orthopedic conditions, including femoral head osteonecrosis. Leg length difference is caused by lumbar spine involvement with osteonecrosis and collapse with subsequent sclerosis. Intraoperative blood loss should be avoided as feasible in patients with a high difficulty score, and blood transfusions should be administered as needed.

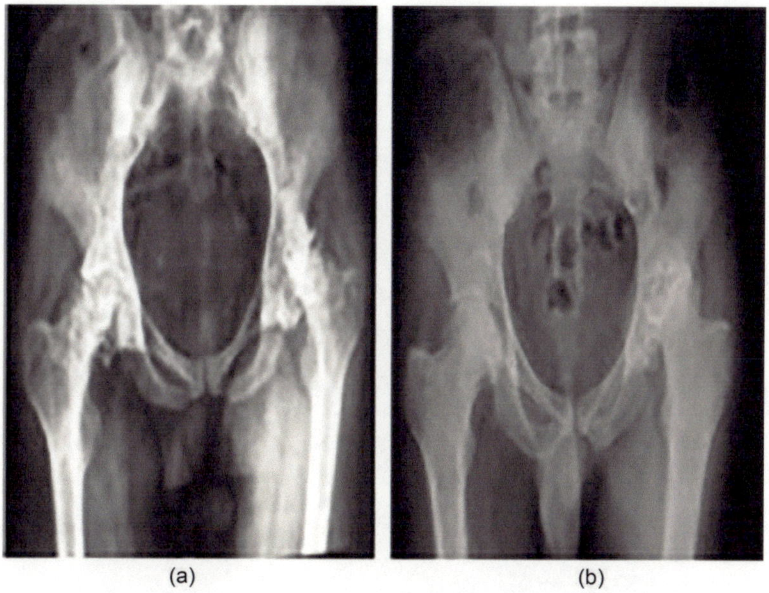

Figure 4.
(a) Advanced bilateral a vascular necrosis away from hips; (b) unilateral a vascular necrosis restricted to the left hip.

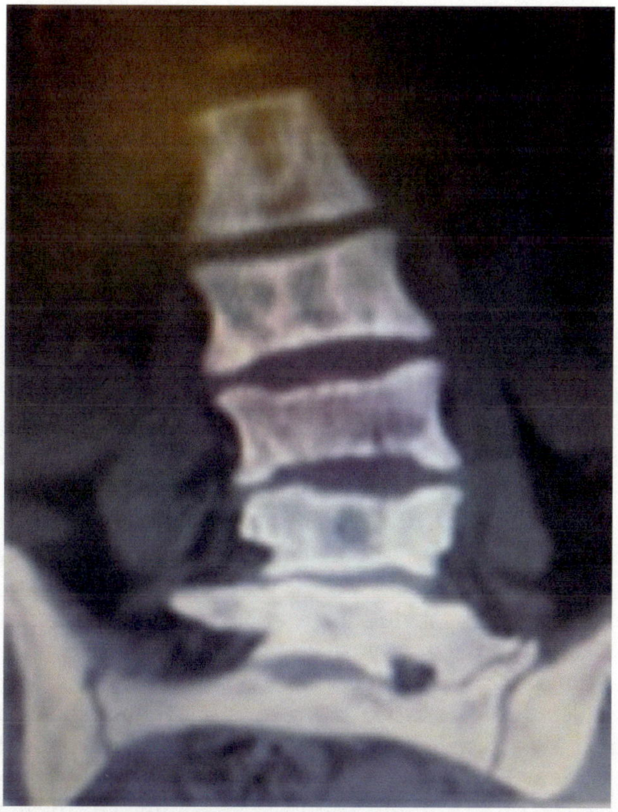

Figure 5.
Scoliosis of the spine secondary to a vascular necrosis.

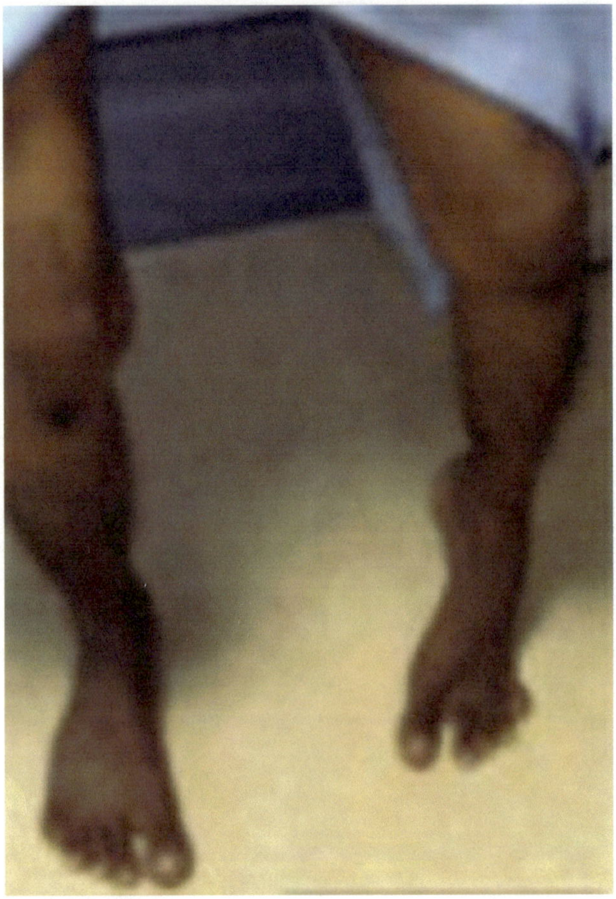

Figure 6.
Soft tissue hip and knee contractures.

Sickle cell anemia is a kind of anemia that affects vascular necrosis, which affects the hip joint early in a patient's life. As sickle cell anemia patients' survival rates improve, it is more likely that hip replacement and revision procedures will be performed sooner than expected [40]. Infarcts cause most instances with boney infarct without loss of congruency with intraosseous compartmental pressure of the femoral head, which may benefit from core decompression [39]. Hips become complicated since the disease has deteriorated owing to weakness, stiffness, and a lack of desire by the time they present.

The time necessary for surgery is equivalent to the time required for a problematic main hip, and our findings are consistent with those of other writers. Technical challenges observed during surgery included the severity of localized disease alterations such as stiffness, femoral canal obliteration, and acetabular bone stock variation due to cysts, sclerosis, and protrusio in rare cases.

Intraoperative blood loss varies according to these technological challenges, necessitating more blood transfusions. Our study's duration is longer than predicted compared with previous studies on primary total hip replacement (THR), which had mean operational times of 89 minutes and 12,328 minutes. The mean intraoperative blood loss was 1600 ml, more significant than the 1090 ml, 984 ml, and about 371 ml reported in primary THR.

The acetabulum of the femur can both be perforated and fractured. The individuals who had femoral perforation did not require any additional treatment. The channel was ultimately discovered, and the stem was able to avoid the hole. A sickler and a young guy with steroid-induced AVN both had acetabular perforation. Due to severe irregularity and a poor acetabular floor, the hole developed during reaming. In sicklers, Al-Mousawi [41] found acetabular perforation, femoral perforation, and fractures identical to our findings.

At birth, the hip joint lacks sphericity and congruency. It is also prone to subluxation and dislocations due to its lack of rigidity. A deeper spherical acetabular cavity occurs due to stress and musculoskeletal alterations, enhancing joint stability [42].

Osteoarthritis of the hip can be caused by various developmental disorders defined by a lack of hip joint congruency. However, femoroacetabular impingements might be a secondary cause of osteoarthritis [43]. Patients with a lack of congruency were thought to have more significant clinical problems, and complete hip replacement in these patients would result in substantial functional benefits.

9. Postoperative care

After surgery, the patients got routine physical therapy for total hip replacement, including pain management, muscle-strengthening activities, patient education, and range of motion. Partially weight-bearing was allowed for the first 6 weeks, followed by full weight-bearing. Ten to twenty-one days after surgery, the patients were discharged from the hospital.

The functional results were assessed using the Harris Hip Score (HHS) [44]. To evaluate functional results clinically and radiographically, all patients were followed up at 6-week intervals and subsequently at 6-month intervals. Loosening, dislocation, and heterotopic ossification were all looked for on radiographs.

Surgical problems, infection, loosening, and dislocation were all considered failures, necessitating revision replacement surgery. Patients were examined by a hematologist and the research author at each follow-up, and medical and surgical problems were recorded.

10. Differential diagnosis

A vascular necrosis of the femoral head symptoms coincides with other etiologies that should be considered in a differential diagnosis. The first is bone marrow edema syndrome (BMES), also known as temporary osteoporosis, which develops due to an accident, increased physical activity, or osteoarthritis. This syndrome manifests as sudden, atraumatic hip discomfort that is self-limited and usually fades within a year (**Table 2**).

Magnetic resonance imaging or extensive bone marrow edema gives the condition its name; imaging is frequently essential [45]. A subchondral fracture, which commonly arises as a fracture following minor trauma in the elderly, in the setting of osteoporosis leading to subchondral insufficiency, is another disorder that can be mistaken with osteonecrosis of the proximal head of the femur.

Complex regional pain syndrome
Inflammatory synovitis
bone marrow edema syndrome (BMES)
Osteomyelitis
Osteoarthritis
Osteoporosis
Soft tissue trauma

Table 2.
Problems faced by patients in osteonecrosis.

11. Prognosis

Many variables influence the prognosis of femoral head osteonecrosis. The point at when it is diagnosed is one of them. The sooner an illness is diagnosed, the more successful the preventative measures are and the better the prognosis.

Moreover, there are markers of a poor prognosis such as lateral head involvement, age > 50 years, and involvement of greater than one-third of the weight-bearing portion of the femoral head, along with the disease advancement when the diagnosis is being made [46]. A patient's prognosis might differ and should be decided by a skilled physician following an adequate examination; although, one or more of these characteristics are present [47].

12. Complications

Joint discomfort worsens with time, decreased range of motion, and osteoarthritis are all complications [48]. Patients may have a considerable handicap as a result of these consequences.

13. Consultations

A trained orthopedic surgeon should be consulted for an expert examination when a practitioner believes a patient has femoral head osteonecrosis.

14. Deterrence and patient education

Patients should seek medical attention if patients are suffering discomfort in their hips, thighs, or buttocks. Specific patient populations should be informed of the risk factors and tested as appropriate because early a vascular necrosis of the femoral head might be asymptomatic.

Patients on long-term steroid treatment, long-term bisphosphonates, heavy alcohol usage, hemoglobinopathies, chemotherapy or radiation patients, and those who sustain damage to the hip and surrounding region are all examples of higher-risk patients [23].

15. Enhancing healthcare team outcomes

Many inter-professional individuals' makeup healthcare teams, including (but not limited to) a physician, nurse practitioner or physician assistant, pharmacist, and nurse. All members of this team who treat patients with a vascular necrosis of the femoral head must recognize the problem, engage in a qualified care plan, and seek expert advice when necessary. The pharmacist can assist in evaluating drug regimens, both in the lead-up to AVN and in attempts to treat AVN pharmaceutically, and can report any concerns to the physician.

If surgery is required, an orthopedic specialist will lead the treatment, and nursing will assist in preparing the patient for surgery, monitoring the patient during and after surgery, and checking on treatment efficacy as well as administering postoperative medications, all while keeping an eye out for adverse effects that should be reported as soon as possible.

Patients should be educated about the dangers of drinking by primary care providers, especially nurses. In addition, doctors should use the lowest effective dosage of corticosteroids when prescribing them. Patients taking long-term corticosteroids should be queried about hip discomfort at every clinic visit by nurses and doctors. The pharmacist should educate patients about the importance of quitting smoking and collaborate with physicians to develop pharmacological aids to help smokers quit. Patients should be educated on the signs and symptoms of AVN to seek treatment as soon as possible.

Each inter-professional healthcare team member's awareness and knowledge of a vascular necrosis of the femoral head will enhance patient treatment and prognosis outcomes.

16. Conclusion

In sickle cell anemia patients, the primary total hip should be adequately prepared; we believe lumping all sickle cell hip a vascular necrosis together is unjust to patients and surgeons. While some of these individuals may be treated with ease, others have a greater degree of difficulty, as evidenced by the existence of musculoskeletal alterations that are not limited to the hip joint.

A thorough history, physical, and radiological examination focusing on these predictors of poor prognosis are required to distinguish between the two groups. Strict preoperative optimization is needed, as well as a well-stocked implant arsenal for hip replacement. Technically, the hips of sickle cell anemia patients with a high difficulty index are complex; challenges should be anticipated and addressed to minimize a high rate of intraoperative problems, increased operation duration, and blood loss. Primary hip replacement in sickle cell disease patients is prevalent and might be challenging to do.

Acknowledgements

The author is thankful to all the associated personnel who contributed for this study by any means.

Conflict of interest

There is no conflict of interest.

Notes/thanks/other declarations

None.

Author details

Mohammed Lafi Al-Otaibi
Department of Orthopedic Surgery, College of Medicine, King Khalid University, Abha, Kingdom of Saudi Arabia

*Address all correspondence to: mlalotaibi@kku.edu.sa

References

[1] Key NS, Derebail VK. Sickle-cell trait: Novel clinical significance. Hematology. American Society of Hematology. Education Program. 2010;**2010**:418-422. DOI: 10.1182/asheducation-2010.1.418

[2] Efie DT, Joseph NF, Yeika EV, Choukem SP. Severely damaged hip joints from a vascular necrosis in a patient with sickle cell trait: Case report. Journal of Blood Disorders and Transfusion. 2017;**8**:2. DOI: 10.4172/2155-9864.1000387

[3] Vaishya R, Agarwal AK, Edomwonyi EO, Vijay V. Musculoskeletal manifestations of sickle cell disease: A review. Cureus. 2015;**7**(10):e358. DOI: 10.7759/cureus.358

[4] Arbab D, König DP. Atraumatic femoral head necrosis in adults: Epidemiology, etiology, diagnosis, and treatment. Deutsches Ärzteblatt International. 2016;**113**:31. DOI: 10.3238/arztebl.2016.0031

[5] Silva Junior GB, Daher ED, Rocha FA. Osteoarticular involvement in sickle cell disease. Revista Brasileira de Hematologia e Hemoterapia. 2012;**34**:156-164

[6] Naik RP, Haywood C Jr. Sickle cell trait diagnosis: clinical and social implications. Hematology. American Society of Hematology. Education Program. 2015;**2015**:160-167. DOI: 10.1182/asheducation-2015.1.160

[7] Perumal JR, Corbett M. A vascular necrosis of the femoral head in sickle cell trait. Rheumatology. 1978;**17**:113. DOI: 10.1093/rheumatology/17.2.113

[8] Houwing ME, de Pagter PJ, van Beers EJ, Biemond BJ, Rettenbacher E, Rijneveld AW, et al. Sickle cell disease: Clinical presentation and management of a global health challenge. Blood Reviews. 2019;**37**:100580. DOI: 10.1016/j.blre.2019.05.004

[9] Yawn BP, Buchanan GR, Afenyi-Annan AN, Ballas SK, Hassell KL, James AH, et al. Management of sickle cell disease: Summary of the 2014 evidence-based report by expert panel members. Journal of the American Medical Association. 2014;**312**:1033-1048. DOI: 10.1001/jama.2014.10517

[10] Al-Otaibi ML, Waliullah S, Kumar V. Total hip replacement in sickle cell disease patients with a vascular necrosis of head of femur: A retrospective observational study. Indian Journal of Orthopaedics. 2021;**28**;55(5):1225-1231. DOI: 10.1007/s43465-021-00394-6

[11] Silva Junior GB, Daher ED, Rocha FA. Osteoarticular involvement in sickle cell disease. Revista Brasileira de Hematologia e Hemoterapia. 2012;**34**:156-164. DOI: 10.5581/1516-8484.20120036

[12] Ilyas I, Alrumaih HA, Rabbani S. Noncemented total hip arthroplasty in sickle-cell disease: Long-term results. The Journal of Arthroplasty. 2018;**33**: 477-481. DOI: 10.1016/j.arth.2017.09.010

[13] Jack CM, Howard J, Aziz ES, Kesse-Adu R, Bankes MJ. Cementless total hip replacements in sickle cell disease. Hip International. 2016;**26**:186-192. DOI: 10.5301/hipint.5000317

[14] Petek D, Hannouche D, Suva D. Osteonecrosis of the femoral head: Pathophysiology and current concepts of treatment. EFORT Open Reviews. 2019;**4**:85-97. DOI: 10.1302/2058-5241.4.180036

[15] Caracalla M, Mair SD. StatPearls [Internet]. Treasure Island (FL): StatPearls Publishing; 2020. p. 20

[16] Narayanan A, Khanchandani P, Borkar RM, Ambati CR, Roy A, Han X, et al. A vascular necrosis of femoral head: A metabolomic, biophysical, biochemical, electron microscopic and histopathological characterization. Scientific Reports. 2017;**7**:1-6. DOI: 10.1038/s41598-017-10817-w

[17] Baig SA, Baig MN. Osteonecrosis of the femoral head: Etiology, investigations, and management. Cureus. 2018;**10**(8):e3171. DOI: 10.7759/cureus.3171

[18] Xie XH, Wang XL, Yang HL, Zhao DW, Qin L. Steroid-associated osteonecrosis: Epidemiology, pathophysiology, animal model, prevention, and potential treatments (an overview). Journal of Orthopaedic Translation. 2015;**3**(2):58-70. DOI: 10.1016/j.jot.2014.12.002

[19] Jaffré C, Rochefort GY. Alcohol-induced osteonecrosis–dose and duration effects. International Journal of Experimental Pathology. 2012;**93**:78. DOI: 10.1111/j.1365-2613.2011.00798_1.x

[20] Adesina O, Brunson A, Keegan TH, Wun T. Osteonecrosis of the femoral head in sickle cell disease: Prevalence, comorbidities, and surgical outcomes in California. Blood Advances. 2017;**1**:1287-1295. DOI: 10.1182/bloodadvances.2017005256

[21] Barney J, Piuzzi NS, Akhondi H. Femoral Head A vascular Necrosis. [Updated 2021 Jul 6]. In: StatPearls [Internet]. Treasure Island (FL): StatPearls Publishing; 2022 Jan-. Available from: https://www.ncbi.nlm.nih.gov/books/NBK546658/

[22] Tripathy SK, Goyal T, Sen RK. Management of femoral head osteonecrosis: Current concepts. Indian Journal of Orthopaedics. 2015;**49**:28-45. DOI: 10.4103/0019-5413.143911

[23] Moya-Angeler J, Gianakos AL, Villa JC, Ni A, Lane JM. Current concepts on osteonecrosis of the femoral head. World Journal of Orthopedics. 2015;**6**:590. DOI: 10.5312/wjo.v6.i8.590

[24] Vardhan H, Tripathy SK, Sen RK, Aggarwal S, Goyal T. Epidemiological profile of femoral head osteonecrosis in the north Indian population. Indian Journal of Orthopaedics. 2018;**52**:140-146

[25] Learmonth ID, Young C, Rorabeck C. The operation of the century: Total hip arthroplasty. Lancet. 2007;**390**: 1508-1519. DOI: 10.1016/s0140-6736(07)60457-7

[26] Evans JT, Evans JP, Walker RW, Blom AW, Whitehouse MR, Sayers A. How long does a hip replacement last? A systematic review and meta-analysis of case series and national registry reports with more than 15 years of follow-up. The Lancet. 2019;**393**:647-654. DOI: 10.1016/s0140-6736(18)31665-9

[27] Kenanidis E, Kapriniotis K, Anagnostis P, Potoupnis M, Christofilopoulos P, Tsiridis E. Total hip arthroplasty in sickle cell disease: A systematic review. EFORT Open Reviews. 2020;**5**:180-188. DOI: 10.1302/2058-5241.5.190038

[28] Vichinsky E, Hoppe CC, Ataga KI, Ware RE, Nduba V, El-Beshlawy A, et al. A phase 3 randomized trial of voxelotor in sickle cell disease. The New England Journal of Medicine. 2019;**381**:509-519. DOI: 10.1056/nejmoa1903212

[29] Autauga KI, Kutlar A, Kanter J, Liles D, Cancado R, Friedrich J, et al.

Crizanlizumab for the prevention of pain crises in sickle cell disease. The New England Journal of Medicine. 2017;**376**:429-439. DOI: 10.1056/nejmoa1611770

[30] Sadaf A, Quinn CT. L-glutamine for sickle cell disease: Knight or pawn? Experimental Biology and Medicine. 2020;**245**:146-154. DOI: 10.1177/1535370219900637

[31] Niihara Y, Miller ST, Kanter J, Lanzkron S, Smith WR, Hsu LL, et al. A phase 3 trial of l-glutamine in sickle cell disease. The New England Journal of Medicine. 2018;**379**:226-235. DOI: 10.1056/nejmoa1715971

[32] de la Fuente J, Gluckman E, Makani J, Telfer P, Faulkner L, Corbacioglu S, et al. The role of hematopoietic stem cell transplantation for sickle cell disease in the era of targeted disease-modifying therapies and gene editing. The Lancet Haematology. 2020;**7**:e902-e911. DOI: 10.1016/s2352-3026(20)30283-0

[33] Robinson TM, Fuchs EJ. Allogeneic stem cell transplantation for sickle cell disease. Current Opinion in Hematology. 2016;**23**:524. DOI: 10.1097/moh.0000000000000282

[34] Erick EB, Lehmann LE, Biffi A, Achebe M, Brendel C, Ciuculescu MF, et al. Post-transcriptional genetic silencing of BCL11A to treat sickle cell disease. The New England Journal of Medicine. 2021;**384**:205-215. DOI: 10.1056/nejmoa2029392

[35] Frangoul H, Altshuler D, Cappellini MD, Chen YS, Domm J, Eustace BK, et al. CRISPR-Cas9 gene editing for sickle cell disease and β-thalassemia. The New England Journal of Medicine. 2021;**384**:252-260. DOI: 10.1056/nejmoa2031054

[36] Piuzzi NS, Chahla J, Schrock JB, LaPrade RF, Pascual-Garrido C, Mont MA, et al. Evidence for the use of cell-based therapy for the treatment of osteonecrosis of the femoral head: A systematic review of the literature. The Journal of Arthroplasty. 2017;**32**:1698-1708. DOI: 10.1016/j.arth.2016.12.049

[37] Piuzzi NS, Chahla J, Jiandong H, Chughtai M, LaPrade RF, Mont MA, et al. Analysis of cell therapies used in clinical trials for the treatment of osteonecrosis of the femoral head: A systematic review of the literature. The Journal of Arthroplasty. 2017;**32**:2612-2618. DOI: 10.1016/j.arth.2017.02.075

[38] Lespasio MJ, Sodhi N, Mont MA. Osteonecrosis of the hip: A primer. The Permanente Journal. 2019;**23**. DOI: 10.7812/tpp/18-100

[39] Al-Otaibi ML. Hip replacement in sickle cell anemia patient and the effect of musculoskeletal changes other than hip joint on outcome. Middle East Journal of Family Medicine. 2021;**7**:20

[40] Sathappan SS, Strauss EJ, Ginat D, Upasani V, Di Cesare PE. Surgical challenges in complex primary total hip arthroplasty. American Journal of Orthopedics. 2007;**36**:534

[41] Al-Mousawi F. Complications and failures of hip replacement in sickle cell disease. Bahrain Medical Bulletin. 2004;**26**:134-138

[42] Giorgi M, Carriero A, Shefelbine SJ, Nowlan NC. Effects of normal and abnormal loading conditions on morphogenesis of the prenatal hip joint: Application to hip dysplasia. Journal of Biomechanics. 2015;**48**:3390-3397. DOI: 10.1016/j.jbiomech.2015.06.002

[43] Ganz R, Leunig M, Leunig-Ganz K, Harris WH. The etiology of osteoarthritis

of the hip. Clinical Orthopaedics and Related Research. 2008;**466**:264-272. DOI: 10.1007/s11999-007-0060-z

[44] Singh JA, Schleck C, Harmsen S, Lewallen D. Clinically important improvement thresholds for Harris hip score and its ability to predict revision risk after primary total hip arthroplasty. BMC Musculoskeletal Disorders. 2016;**17**:1-8. DOI: 10.1186/s12891-016-1106-8

[45] Choi HR, Steinberg ME, Cheng EY. Osteonecrosis of the femoral head: Diagnosis and classification systems. Current Reviews in Musculoskeletal Medicine. 2015;**8**:210-220. DOI: 10.1007/s12178-015-9278-7

[46] Goker B, Block JA. Risk of contralateral a vascular necrosis (AVN) after total hip arthroplasty (THA) for non-traumatic AVN. Rheumatology International. 2006;**26**:215-219. DOI: 10.1007/s00296-004-0554-x

[47] Niimi R, Sudo A, Hasegawa M, Uchida A. Course of a vascular necrosis of femoral head without collapse of femoral head at first examination: Minimum 8-year follow-up. Orthopedics. 2008;**31**:755

[48] Hauzeur JP, De Maertelaer V, Baudoux E, Malaise M, Beguin Y, Gangji V. Inefficacy of autologous bone marrow concentrate in stage three osteonecrosis: A randomized controlled double-blind trial. International Orthopaedics. 2018;**42**:1429-1435. DOI: 10.1007/s00264-017-3650-8

Chapter 2

Digital Health Interventions to Empower People with Sickle Cell Disease: Toward Patient-Led Design

David-Zacharie Issom

Abstract

This chapter will provide a state of the art of digital health interventions for people with sickle cell disease. It will use WHO classification of digital health interventions to elaborate on existing intervention, the gaps, and how technology could be useful to support people with sickle cell disease. A description of the existing possibilities, the current trends, and the future opportunities will be provided. As well, methodologies to increase patient adherence to digital health interventions, the importance of participatory approaches, open innovation, and patient-led approaches to designing such interventions will be discussed. Importantly, a holistic/planetary health approach will be chosen to introduce the subject and ensure to keep a broad eye on the domain and to include sustainability challenges.

Keywords: digital health interventions, artificial intelligence, self-management, integrated care, patient empowerment, participatory design

1. Introduction

Sickle cell disease (SCD) is the world's most common monogenic pathology. SCD is a complex multisystem red blood cell disorder, which leads many patients to experience acute life-threatening dysfunctions and chronic complications. The hallmarks of the disease are vaso-occlusive pain crises (VOCs), avascular necrosis, hemolytic anemia, endothelial dysfunction, transient ischemic attacks, acute chest syndrome (ACS), bacterial infections, and chronic inflammation. These complications cause reduced Health-Related Quality of Life (HRQoL) and increased mortality [1].

To limit complications and reduce early mortality, integrated care, also known as comprehensive and coordinated care (CPC), is paramount. Indeed, CPC has demonstrated efficacy in improving health outcomes of people affected by multisystemic diseases such as diabetes [2]. In the case of SCD, CPC shall cover different forms of care provision, including acute care (e.g., treatment of VOCs), usual care, defined as routine evaluations and treatments (e.g., transcranial Doppler testing), chronic transfusion therapies, or disease-modifying treatments (e.g., hydroxyurea) [3].

The latter treatments remain underutilized and limited [4]. Access to curative options (e.g., hematopoietic stem-cell transplantations, gene therapy) remains restrained [5]. As well, specific comprehensive and preventative care (CPC) programs are inconsistently available for most people with SCD [6]. Consequently, many patients do not receive adequate treatment, as outlined by evidence-based guidelines, and may suffer from mistrust, stigmatization, or neglect [7].

As a result, patients must rely heavily on themselves and their community to manage symptoms, maintain control over the course of the disease, and preserve an acceptable level of Health-Related Quality of Life (HRQoL) [4, 8]. Because of its complexity, SCD self-management can be particularly challenging to master [9]. Indeed, self-management covers various aspects, ranging from self-care in hospitalization, post-hospitalization care, hospital-at-home care, preventive care, health maintenance, or self-care aspects such as self-monitoring, self-diagnosis, self-treatment [10, 11].

For instance, every day, patients should take prescribed drugs, follow a healthy diet, hydrate frequently, avoid strenuous exercise, check indicators of anemia, which could manifest by increased pallor, dark urine color, or jaundice. As well, patients should observe warning signs of complications, monitor and treat their chronic or acute pain with prescribed medication and other nondrug therapies (e.g., breathing exercise, physical therapy, phytotherapy), or pay attention to numerous and omnipresent potential precipitants of VOCs [9, 10].

Such triggers include certain food, stress, infections, acidosis, dehydration, fatigue, hypoxia, alcohol intoxication, daytime exertion, exercise, airline travel, altitude, pregnancy, nocturnal hypoxemia, or environmental factors including pollution, exposure to the elements, change of temperatures, wind, or humidity [12–15]. The quantity and complexity of these factors demands autonomy, resilience, high self-efficacy, and empowerment levels, as well as adequate psychosocial support [16, 17].

Due to their socioeconomic positions, most patients lack such skills and consequently adherence to recommended treatments, self-care recommendations, or attendance to routine clinic appointments (RCA) remains low [18]. However, some patients have proven to be exceptions. As long-term users of healthcare services, some acquired knowledge that made them efficient navigators of healthcare systems, while gaining singular expertise in self-management, succeeding to learn how they could improve their HRQoL [19, 20].

As Ballas et al. [20] pointed out, these strongly equipped patients succeeded to identify their own best self-care practices or became able to notice and react to warning signs from their body. Some would journal their symptoms, manage their pain successfully, follow adequate dietary habits, practice moderate physical activity, or attend RCA [21, 22].

The complex nature of SCD such as a high individual and population variability, or a rising number of people affected due to lack of systematic screening, poor awareness about the disease or migrations of populations [23], its scientific and social history, its high economic burden, and the diversity of the endogenous and exogenous factors combining to influence health outcomes (e.g., multifaceted health disparities, stigma, racism, underfunding) require researchers and policymakers to take care of SCD through various lenses [24].

For all these reasons, it appears particularly relevant and urgent to investigate cost-effective and easily scalable interventional strategies to prevent serious complications, avoid hospitalizations, and more generally, empower and improve the quality of life of people with SCD.

2. Strategies to empower people with SCD

Given SCD global burden, the complexity, and number of challenges to be overcome (e.g., neglect, continuous rise, stigma, underfunding) [25–29], it is important to prioritize effective interventions and shorten the timeframe for action. Fortunately, after the great advances in the 1970s (e.g., American civil rights organizations promised to vote for the future President Nixon if policies and funding were put in place to counter SCD), FDA approval of Hydroxyurea in 1995 [30], repeated calls to action during the last couple of years and recent advances in genomics [26–28, 31], SCD has been increasingly regarded as an interesting model to study and address from different angles in particular since 2017 [32–39]. This renewed interest opens hope that research advances could enable possibilities of generalization, reutilization, and transfer to other NCDs, while subsequently empowering more populations and enhancing life opportunities.

To move forward in a coordinated manner, and to effectively shape health and social policies aiming at empowering underserved populations, global health agents need a clear strategy, a unified agenda, and a strong commitment with the adequate resources. To proceed, the American National Academy of Sciences [40], the WHO, and various scholars have proposed priority targets for SCD [4, 26, 41–44].

These recommendations range from installing national surveillance programs, promoting better use of disease-modifying treatments, increasing the funding of disease-specific research, raising awareness, improving pain relief management, tackling systemic violence (e.g., stigma, racism), improving training for healthcare providers, increasing the numbers of specialists, promoting access to comprehensive and preventative care, empowering communities, creating therapeutic education programs, supporting self-care management, and encouraging the use of Information and Communication Technologies (ICTs) [4, 26, 41, 42].

3. Digitalization as a lever to reduce health inequalities

As research suggests (e.g., health impact pyramid), interventions that could empower as many individuals as possible should be prioritized [45, 46]. Today, as the International Telecommunication Union (ITU) illustrates [47], Information and Communications Technologies (ICTs), thanks to their increasingly important presence in people's daily lives (e.g., smartphones, smart sensors), could play major roles in driving rapid social transformation, empowering populations from their social determinisms, and accelerating the achievement of challenges of the centuries such as the Sustainable Development Goals (SDGs) [48].

Recent years have seen the rise of digital technologies in the healthcare sector (e.g., computerized drug prescription systems reducing risks of medical errors, remote surgery, early detection of seizures or heart failures) [49]. To achieve most vital SDGs such as *no poverty, no hunger, good health and well-being,* exploring the potential of digital health technologies seems particularly relevant to empower people with SCD and reduce the health inequality gap.

As the WHO acknowledged, thanks to their potential to be scaled up rapidly to reach large numbers of people, digital technologies hold the potential to accelerate a decline in health inequalities through disease-specific actions [50].

Notably, stressing the importance of ensuring that such tools provide an evidence-based improvement in health outcomes, the WHO emphasizes that *such interventions should (i) complement and (ii) enhance health system functions through the acceleration of the exchange of information, (iii) improve access to healthcare, (iv) be affordable, and (v) should not replace the fundamental components needed by health systems, such as the health workforce, financing, leadership and governance, or access to medicines* [50].

The following sections describe WHO's classification of digital health interventions (DHIs) and illustrate what specific DHI characteristics might support SCD-important challenges [51].

4. Digital health interventions

In the context of low availability of specialized healthcare service and thanks to potential wide reach and relatively low cost, digital health interventions (DHIs) could offer a potential route to help patients become experts in self-management [52–55].

As per WHO definition, digital health encompasses various concepts including eHealth (i.e., effective use of information and communication for health-related purposes), mHealth (i.e., provision of information and services through mobile technologies), or telemedicine (i.e., remote practice of medical interventions or examination) [56–58]. Additionally, digital health includes computing techniques (e.g., artificial intelligence, natural language processing, interoperability), which assist in extracting and making sense of a large volume of health-related data (e.g., genomic sequencing, medical imaging, health records, medical devices, wearables, pharmaceutical research, search engines, online patient communities, healthcare payor records) [59, 60]. Health interventions using digital technologies can be classified in four categories, based on the targeted primary user.

Overall, DHIs are increasingly used to provide effective, safe, and scalable interventions improving chronic patient's health outcomes [61]. However, prior studies found that patients who stand to benefit most from DHIs were least likely to download or use them [62, 63]. With discontinued or inconsistent use, it is less likely that the intended effectiveness of DHIs can be realized.

Studies have shown that DHIs responding effectively to patients' specific health problems while being easy to use had better long-term engagement [64, 65]. Interestingly, Stenft et al. [66] demonstrated that engagement in DHIs was higher among patients who were dissatisfied with healthcare service delivery (HSD). Additionally, Lee et al. [67] suggested that these patients particularly desired to get access to novel technologies and would request specific digital health services keeping them away from hospitals. As prior studies suggest [68–70], including patients' input from the start to the end of design, development and evaluation phases could help creating DHIs that are desired, used, and engaging in the long run.

The potential of digital health technologies for SCD is far from being fully exploited, and patients' experiential knowledge is largely untapped. Indeed, most DHIs focus on symptom monitoring or medication adherence [71]. However, given the multisystemic nature of SCD, its multiple vulnerability factors, its clinical variability, and severe comorbidities, it is paramount to encompass every components of self-management and to comprehensively support the day-to-day and long-term self-care needs of patients.

5. Categories of digital health interventions

5.1 Category 1: interventions for clients

The first category defines interventions for clients, i.e., individuals such as patients, citizens, or informal caregivers. The aim of such DHIs ranges from improving access to care for remote populations, disseminating targeted education to providers and patients through eHealth, and supporting patient empowerment with mHealth self-management apps targeting smoking cessation, medication dosage calculators, support for medication adherence, symptoms self-monitoring, or remote medical consultations, see **Figure 1**. For instance, Jacob et al.recently demonstrated how telemedicine could help deliver CPC to remote children with SCD in underserved areas [72].

Today, mHealth apps are flooding app stores, with more than 200 new apps each day, and a sharp rise during the COVID-19 outbreak [73–75]. Many of these apps can significantly improve health outcomes and support people with diverse medical conditions [54, 76].

In the case of SCD, some of the existing DHIs could be those that play a role in targeting individual behavioral factors, which are known to cause more than 35% of premature death and are responsible for a large proportion of disease burden [77]. For instance, DHIs could be greatly adapted to help reduce knowledge-based inequalities among individuals with SCD (e.g., support therapeutic education and self-management, disseminate disease-specific knowledge), or those that could improve awareness about the disease. Several authors have demonstrated tools to support

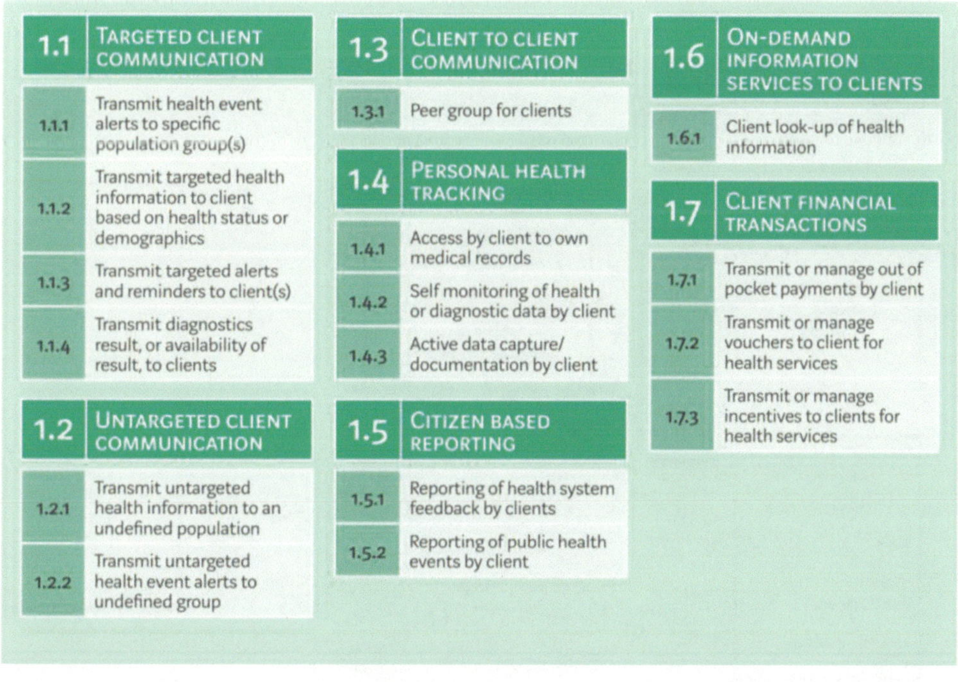

Figure 1.
Digital health interventions for clients—WHO [51].

mental health among people with SCD. Some systems utilize text-based technology to conduct psychological interventions [78], while others propose effective ways to conduct cognitive behavioral therapy remotely using mobile apps [79].

As **Figure 2** illustrates [8], self-care elements of disease management are particularly important when designing mHealth apps targeting patients. Indeed, because good self-care practices lead to positive health outcomes, DHIs, thanks to their relatively low cost and wide reach, could be a potential route to support people with SCD's numerous self-care management tasks, for instance, by improving their health literacy or increasing their self-efficacy levels [80–82].

Findings from multiple studies have identified an increasing number of digital health interventions aiming to support people with SCD [39, 71, 83]. However, the potential of digital health technologies for people with SCD is far from being fully exploited but has started to accelerate in the recent years. Indeed, most DHIs focus on symptom monitoring or medication adherence, but promising studies described how self-management mHealth apps could enhance patient engagement in disease management [71, 84, 85]. Although not comprehensive, this study provides useful evidence on the needs and wants of adults with SCD.

However, similar to other chronic diseases, the frequency of downloads and long-term adoption remains in its infancy [84]. In an attempt to tackle such an important issue, Philips et al. [86] and Issom et al. [87] proposed to put more efforts in the direction of patient-centered and patient-led approaches when designing digital health interventions, so we can better understand factors encouraging adoption [88]. Authors suggested methodologies such as the Behavior Change Wheel to understand human and societal factors important to take into account to reach higher rates of appreciation and increased motivation in using DHIs by patients [89].

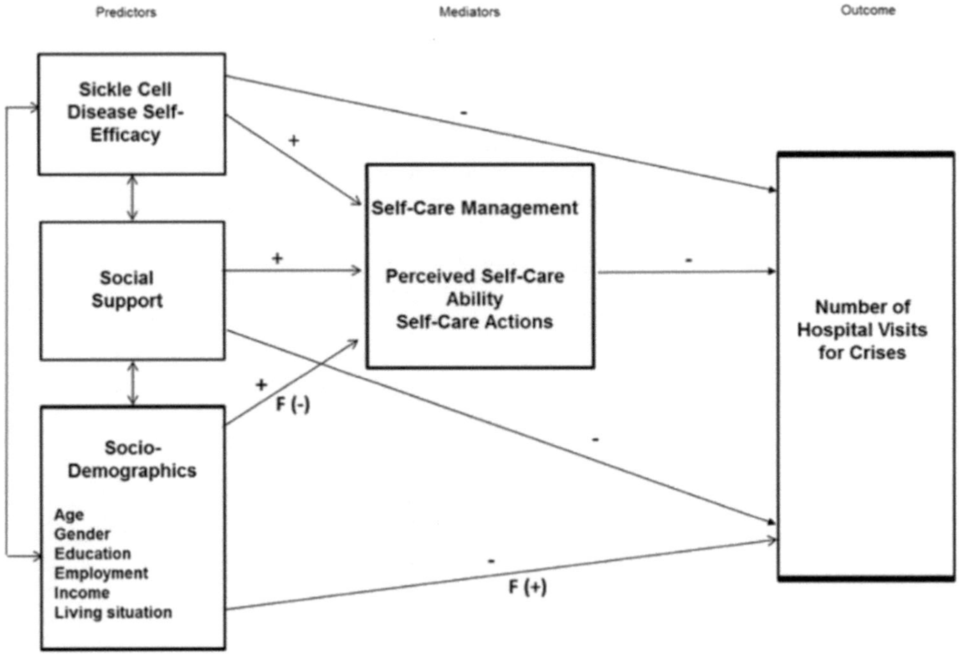

Figure 2.
Role of self-care in sickle cell disease—Matthie et al. [8].

As well, authors suggested the use of systems using lower energetical resources and easy to learn (e.g., chatbots) to foster adherence and reduce costs. Still, more research is needed and important patient-important needs (e.g., reduce the incidence of pains, self-care support, improve self-efficacy, increase disease-specific knowledge, support transition to adulthood) are yet to be tackled effectively [90, 91], but existing research studies are encouraging, showing potential in increasing important these important outcomes [92–94]. Johnson et al. [95] demonstrated the feasibility of an innovative way to mitigate pain crises by using wearable devices signals to monitor pain and attempt at predicting symptoms using machine learning approaches. Similarly, Ajayi et al.showed how such systems could be used to collect a wide range of biophysical measurements [96]. Yet, today, most apps for people with SCD reported in the scientific literature focus on medication adherence or the monitoring of symptoms [71, 84]. Hankins and Shah analyzed the matter and the importance of adherence and proposed a framework to tackle medication adherence using mobile apps [97].

5.2 Category 2: interventions for healthcare providers

Research is scarce regarding DHIs for healthcare providers specialized in SCD [98]. Nevertheless, such digital health interventions could be helpful in supporting the scarcity of healthcare professionals specialized in SCD care. As **Figure 3** illustrates, the WHO promotes the development of tools such as micro-learning apps for healthcare provider training, decision support systems, or infrastructure for remote consultations. Such DHIs hold the potential to increase the pool of specialized healthcare providers, improve patient-provider communication, or coordinate care. Researchers have investigated tools to improve medical decision-making, for instance, by providing guidance on pain management and curative treatment [98, 99] or by supporting diagnostic of sickle cell disease using digital PCR or mobile microscopy [100, 101].

5.3 Category 3: interventions for health systems or resource managers

In the case of SCD, DHIs for health systems managers (**Figure 4**) could be very useful to support the collection of populational epidemiological data (i.e., civil registration, mortality and morbidity data, geographical prevalence) and public health policies to provide patients with targeted support. As well, such DHIs could be helpful in monitoring the quality of SCD care. Today, advances in specific DHIs to help manage disease-specific logistics (e.g., blood products, oxygen tanks, epidemiological data) or to provide targeted information to clinicians susceptible to encounter people with SCD (e.g., clinical guidelines, emergency protocols, screening equipment) are lacking.

5.4 Category 4: interventions for data services

Data management is a crucial but challenging aspect of DHIs. As **Figure 5** illustrates, DHIs for data services could benefit global health by (1) allowing patients to own their health data; (2) developing robust governance processes that ensure respect of values and principles in the use of data and risk minimization; (3) creating systems that allow for automated collection and aggregation of data; (4) implementing data interoperability standards; (5) allowing anonymized data sharing in real time; and,

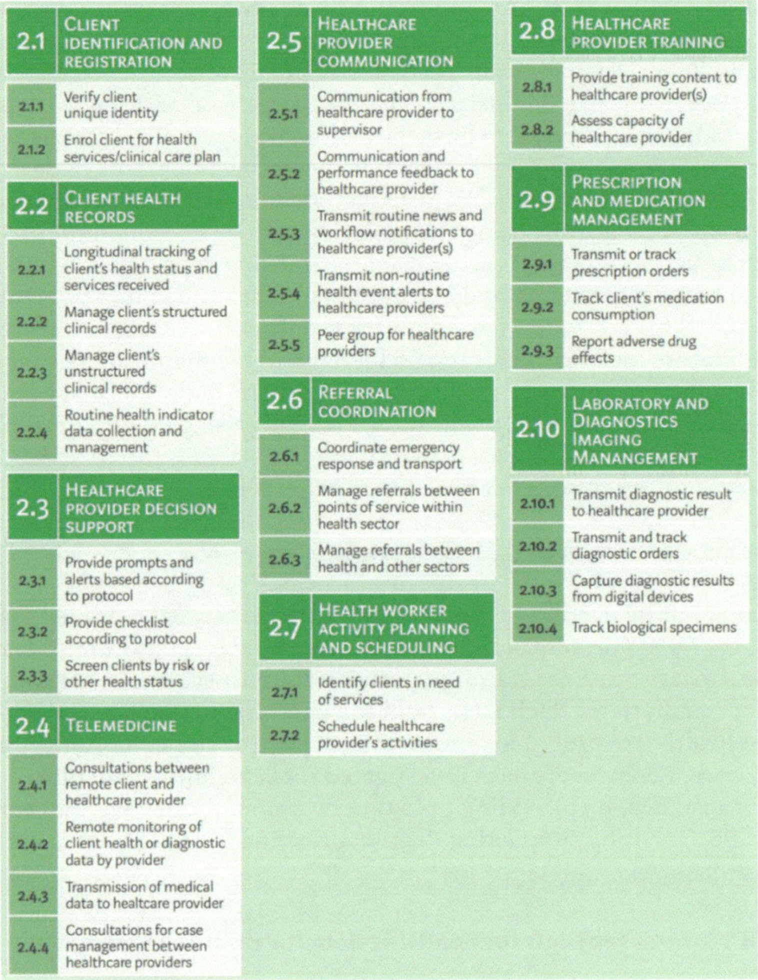

Figure 3.
Digital health interventions for healthcare providers—WHO [51].

(6) formatting and representing data so that they can be easily used by patients, healthcare providers, entrepreneurs, or policymakers [102].

In the case of SCD, DHIs could be crucial to foster the establishment of national data collection of burden of SCD. DHIs focusing on information management could involve supporting national disease surveillance programs, collecting of mortality and morbidity incidences, synthesizing PROMS, analyzing forecasting (e.g., health outcomes, prevalence), and mapping of socioeconomic assistance to the SCD population or promote the creation of health data cooperatives (e.g., databases owned, partly financed, and controlled by the people who use it) [103–105].

6. Structural barriers to the effectiveness of digital health interventions

Setting up effective, sustained, and globally scalable digital health interventions that can contribute to the reduction of disparities is challenging. DHI projects often

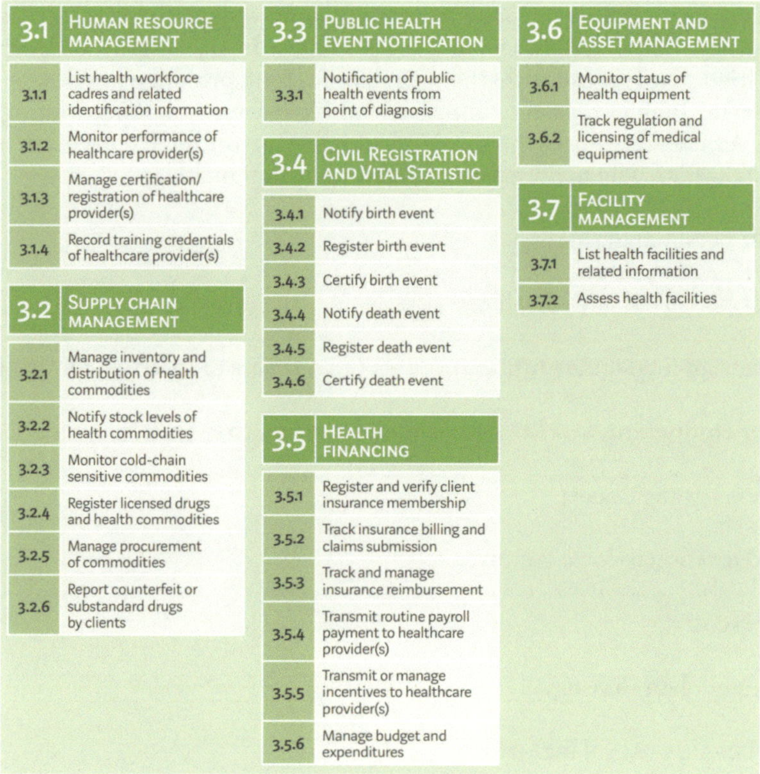

Figure 4.
Digital health interventions for health system managers—WHO [51].

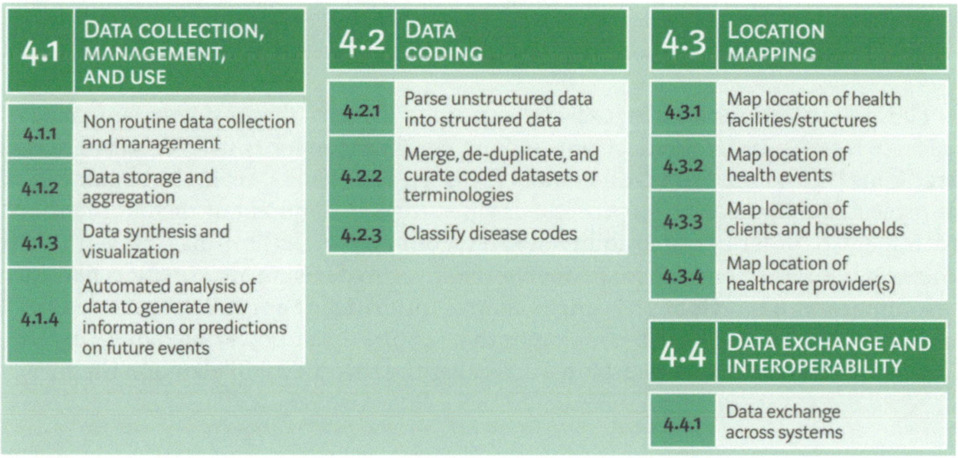

Figure 5.
Digital health interventions for data services—WHO [51].

struggle to scale up sufficiently and are often unsustainable for targeted communities once donor funding ceases [106]. As a result, some projects succeed in transforming the lives of those who have been able to access the technologies, while also disadvantaging those without access to them [107]. Consequently, the number of successfully implemented digital interventions that move beyond the pilot or feasibility stage remains limited. Equally, if and when they pass these initial stages [108], scholars have identified that few users use the technologies for a prolonged period of time, despite offering high potential to improve health outcomes and empowering patients [109–112]. As a result, those who would most benefit from such apps often underuse them [63, 112–124]. The main reasons for low adoption include:

1. lack of personalization;
2. lack of perceived added value;
3. deficient or inadequate infrastructures (e.g., access to Internet connectivity);
4. lack of equipment, low literacy (e.g., digital, health);
5. technology gap issues;
6. maladaptation to local context;
7. hidden costs;
8. unwanted data sharing;
9. insufficiently useful features;
10. inability to sustain required attention for longer periods of time;
11. financial unsustainability;
12. poor usability (e.g., suboptimal design, manual data entry) [113, 125–128].

These observations may partially be explained using such top-down approaches to design interventions and decision-making. Similarly, in more user-centered design paradigms [120], end users are generally included as partners, from the beginning of the project, during the design process, or when the development of the intervention is complete, in order to test usability or safety, but not as decision-makers. With these processes, i.e., when end users are not contributing to decision-making, it is likely that their important interests are not put as central, prioritized, nor fully acknowledged. Subsequently, this results in technologies that may be disempowering, alienating, or irrelevant to the end users, therefore increasing the risk they will abandon them.

7. People with neglected diseases: from technology enthusiasts to patient innovators

Individuals with orphan diseases and affected by diabetes have been leaders in fostering these approaches using crowdsourcing (i.e., individuals of varying knowledge and skills voluntarily undertaking a task for mutual benefit) or crowdsensing techniques (i.e. using smartphones to sense, collect, and analyze data) to accelerate knowledge discovery and promote patient empowerment [129, 130].

The most famous patient-led innovations are PatientsLikeMe (i.e., the first online community for people with Amyotrophic lateral sclerosis), the #WeAreNotWaiting and #OpenAPS movements (i.e., do-it-yourself methods for creating an artificial pancreas system) [131], the Nightscout project (i.e., a parent-developed solution for remote blood glucose monitoring), or the Crohnology project (e.g., an online platform for patient-to-patient information sharing).

These projects have rapidly reached high number of users, some of them have been acquired by companies in order to ensure financial sustainability or scale-up [132]. These early success stories highlight the importance of user-driven initiatives in research and development and show high potential for patient empowerment [133].

8. Disparate evidence

In June 2019, the WHO and the Organization for Economic Co-operation and Development (OECD) from the European Commission (CE) supported PLR approaches, concluding that digital health interventions should be designed to meet the needs of people and health systems and suit local contexts [134]. Aligned with these conclusions, bottom-up models such as PLR or the free innovation paradigm are becoming increasingly popular [135, 136], exemplifying how researchers in academia, industry, and patient communities can create patient-centric solutions and reduce the disease burden together. Only a few PLR initiatives are mentioned in the scientific literature about SCD, suggesting that most DHIs have been driven by healthcare professionals of software implementers [39, 71]. With their potential of being implemented and scaled up rapidly globally when adequately implemented [137–139], DHIs targeting people with SCD may hold the capacity to address various health inequalities faced by historically disadvantaged populations.

9. Conclusions

Digital health interventions to empower with sickle cell disease remain relatively scarce if we look at their number compared with diseases with higher prevalence, but current research shows a strong potential for improving health outcomes. The important aspects to work on are the human factors allowing a strong adhesion in its interventions and to seek to better understand how to use artificial intelligence to lead to the prediction of symptoms and then to prevent them.

Conflict of interest

The author declare no conflict of interest.

Notes/thanks/other declarations

Place any other declarations, such as "Notes," "Thanks," etc., before the References section. Assign the appropriate heading. Do NOT put your short biography in this section. It will be removed.

Author details

David-Zacharie Issom
Division of Medical Information Sciences, Geneva University Hospitals, Geneva, Switzerland

*Address all correspondence to: david.issom@hcuge.ch

References

[1] Piel FB, Steinberg MH, Rees DC. Sickle cell disease. New England Journal of Medicine. 2017;**376**:1561-1573

[2] Grosse SD, Schechter MS, Kulkarni R, et al. Models of comprehensive multidisciplinary care for individuals in the United States with genetic disorders. Pediatrics. 2009;**123**:407-412

[3] Sandhu MK, Cohen A. Aging in sickle cell disease: Co-morbidities and new issues in management. Hemoglobin. 2015;**39**:221-224

[4] Kanter J, Kruse-Jarres R. Management of sickle cell disease from childhood through adulthood. Blood Reviews. 2013;**27**:279-287

[5] Leonard A, Tisdale J, Abraham A. Curative options for sickle cell disease: Haploidentical stem cell transplantation or gene therapy? British Journal of Haematology. 2020;**189**(3):408-423. DOI: 10.1111/bjh.16437

[6] de Montalembert M. Current strategies for the management of children with sickle cell disease. Expert Review of Hematology. 2009;**2**:455-463

[7] Haywood C, Lanzkron S, Bediako S, et al. Perceived discrimination, patient trust, and adherence to medical recommendations among persons with sickle cell disease. Journal of General Internal Medicine. 2014;**29**:1657-1662

[8] Matthie N, Jenerette C, McMillan S. Role of self-care in sickle cell disease. Pain Management Nursing: Official Journal of the American Society of Pain Management Nurses. 2015;**16**:257-266

[9] Blakemore S. Self-care is key in sickle-cell disease. Emergency Nurse: The Journal of the RCN Accident and Emergency Nursing Association. 2016;**24**:9

[10] Jenerette CM, Brewer C, Leak AN. Self-Care recommendations of middle-aged and older adults with sickle cell disease. Nursing Research and Practice. 2011 Aug 15;**2011**:e270594

[11] Brown S-E, Weisberg DF, Balf-Soran G, et al. Sickle cell disease patients with and without extremely high hospital use: Pain, opioids, and coping. Journal of Pain and Symptom Management. 2015;**49**:539-547

[12] Ahmadi M, Jahani S, Poormansouri S, et al. The Effectiveness of self management program on quality of life in patients with sickle cell disease. Iranian Journal of Pediatric Hematology and Oncology. 2015;**5**:18-26

[13] Norris SL, Engelgau MM, Venkat Narayan KM. Effectiveness of self-management training in type 2 diabetes: A systematic review of randomized controlled trials. Diabetes Care. 2001;**24**:561-587

[14] Jenerette CM, Lauderdale G. Successful aging with sickle cell disease: Using qualitative methods to inform theory. Journal of Theory Construction & Testing. 2008;**12**:16-24

[15] Jenerette CM, Leak AN, Sandelowski M. Life stories of older adults with sickle cell disease. The ABNF Journal: Official Journal of the Association of Black Nursing Faculty in Higher Education, Inc. 2011;**22**:58-63

[16] Mora MA, Luyckx K, Sparud-Lundin C, et al. Patient empowerment in young persons with

chronic conditions: Psychometric properties of the Gothenburg Young Persons Empowerment Scale (GYPES). PLoS One. 2018;**13**:e0201007

[17] Molter BL, Abrahamson K. Self-efficacy, transition, and patient outcomes in the sickle cell disease population. Pain Management Nursing: Official Journal of the American Society of Pain Management Nurses. 2015;**16**:418-424

[18] Cecilio SG, Pereira SA d S, Pinto V d S, et al. Barriers experienced in self-care practice by young people with sickle cell disease. Hematology, Transfusion and Cell Therapy. 2018;**40**:207-212

[19] Kanter J, Issom D-Z. Mind Over Matter: One Person's Journey From Patient to Change-Maker. 2018. Available from: Thehematologist/Profiles/8892.aspx [Accessed: October 17, 2018]

[20] Ballas SK. Self-management of sickle cell disease: A new frontier. Journal of the National Medical Association. 2010;**102**:1042-1043

[21] Amertil NP. Self-management in Adult Clients with Sickle Cell Disease (SCD). 1997. Available from: http://books.google.se/books/about/Self_management_in_Adult_Clients_with_Si.html?id=H-HdtgAACAAJ&pgis=1 [Accessed: September 24, 2014]

[22] Cordeiro RC, Ferreira SL, Santos AC d C, et al. Experiences of illness among individuals with sickle cell anemia and self-care strategies. Acta Paulista de Enfermagem. 2014;**27**:499-504

[23] Royal CDM, Babyak M, Shah N, et al. Sickle cell disease is a global prototype for integrative research and healthcare. Advanced Genetics. 2021;**2**:e10037

[24] Berghs M, Ola B, Chavez ACD, et al. Time to apply a social determinants of health lens to addressing sickle cell disorders in sub-Saharan Africa. BMJ Global Health. 2020;**5**:e002601

[25] Grosse SD, Odame I, Atrash HK, et al. Sickle cell disease in Africa: A neglected cause of early childhood mortality. American Journal of Preventive Medicine. 2011;**41**:S398-S405

[26] Lopez AD, Williams TN, Levin A, et al. Remembering the forgotten non-communicable diseases. BMC Medicine. 2014;**12**:200

[27] Piel FB, Weatherall DJ. Sickle-cell disease: A call to action. Transactions of the Royal Society of Tropical Medicine and Hygiene. 2015;**109**:355-356

[28] Carroll CP. Sickle cell disease: Time to act. Pain Management. 2011;**1**:291-293

[29] Chakravorty S, Williams TN. Sickle cell disease: A neglected chronic disease of increasing global health importance. Archives of Disease in Childhood. 2015;**100**:48-53

[30] Siddiqi A-E-A, Jordan LB, Parker CS. Sickle cell disease—The American Saga. Ethnicity & Disease. 2013;**23**:245-248

[31] Executive Board 117. Executive Board 117th session, Geneva, 23-27 January 2006: Resolutions and decisions, annexes [Internet]. Geneva: World Health Organization; 2006. Available from: https://apps.who.int/iris/handle/10665/20686

[32] Leonard A, Tisdale JF. A pause in gene therapy: Reflecting on the unique challenges of sickle cell disease. Molecular Therapy. 2021;**29**:1355-1356

[33] Salinas Cisneros G, Thein SL. Recent advances in the treatment of sickle cell disease. Frontiers in Physiology. 2020;**11**. DOI: 10.3389/fphys.2020.00435/full

[34] Brodsky RA, DeBaun MR. Are genetic approaches still needed to cure sickle cell disease? The Journal of Clinical Investigation. 2020;**130**:7-9

[35] Carden MA, Little J. Emerging disease-modifying therapies for sickle cell disease. Haematologica. 2019;**104**:1710-1719

[36] Oniyangi O, Cohall DH. Phytomedicines (medicines derived from plants) for sickle cell disease. Cochrane Database of Systematic Reviews (Online). 2015 Jan;**4**:CD004448

[37] Imaga NA. Phytomedicines and nutraceuticals: Alternative therapeutics for sickle cell anemia. The Scientific World Journal. 2013;**2013**:e269659

[38] Williams H, Tanabe P. Sickle cell disease: A review of nonpharmacological approaches for pain. Journal of Pain and Symptom Management. 2016;**51**:163-177

[39] Lobitz S, Curtis K, Sostmann K. Digital Health Interventions (DHIs) to Support the Management of Children and Adolescents with Sickle-Cell Disease. In: Curtis K, editor. Sickle Cell Disease [Internet]. Rijeka: IntechOpen; 2016 [cited 2022 Aug 17]. p. Ch. 14. Available from: https://doi.org/10.5772/64315

[40] Martinez RM, Osei-Anto HA, McCormick M. Summary Table of Strategic Plan and Blueprint for Sickle Cell Disease Action. Addressing Sickle Cell Disease: A Strategic Plan and Blueprint for Action. National Academies Press (US); 2020 Available from: https://www.ncbi.nlm.nih.gov/books/NBK566458/

[41] Aygun B, Odame I. A global perspective on sickle cell disease. Pediatric blood & cancer. 2012;**59**:386-390

[42] Kanter J, Smith WR, Desai PC, et al. Building access to care in adult sickle cell disease: Defining models of care, essential components, and economic aspects. Blood Advances. 2020;**4**:3804-3813

[43] Regional Committee for Africa 60. Sickle-Cell Disease: A strategy for the WHO African Region. 2011. Available from: https://apps.who.int/iris/handle/10665/1682 [Accessed: June 2, 2021]

[44] National Academies of Sciences E. Addressing Sickle Cell Disease: A Strategic Plan and Blueprint for Action. 2020. Available from: https://www.nap.edu/catalog/25632/addressing-sickle-cell-disease-a-strategic-plan-and-blueprint-for [Accessed: June 2, 2021]

[45] Naik A, Bagga S, Sénécal M. PBI15 economic burden of sickle cell disease: A targeted global literature review. Value in Health. 2019;**22**:S420

[46] Lee S, Vania DK, Bhor M, et al. Patient-reported outcomes and economic burden of adults with sickle cell disease in the United States: A systematic review. International Journal of General Medicine. 2020;**13**:361-377

[47] ITU. ICTs to achieve the United Nations Sustainable Development Goals. ITU News. 2018. Available from: https://news.itu.int/icts-united-nations-sustainable-development-goals/ [Accessed: June 30, 2021]

[48] Postcapitalism | Paul Mason | Macmillan. US Macmillan. Available from: https://us.macmillan.com/postcapitalism/paulmason/9780374536732 [Accessed: May 27, 2021]

[49] FDA. What is Digital Health?. FDA. FDA; 2020. Available from: https://www.fda.gov/medical-devices/digital-health-center-excellence/what-digital-health [Accessed: June 17, 2021]

[50] WHO | WHO Guideline: Recommendations on digital interventions for health system strengthening [Internet]. WHO. World Health Organization; 2019 [cited 2020 Jun 17]. Available from: http://www.who.int/reproductivehealth/publications/digital-interventions-health-system-strengthening/en/

[51] WHO. Classification of digital health interventions v1.0 / A shared language to describe the uses of digital technology for health. World Health Organization; 2018. Available from: http://www.who.int/reproductivehealth/publications/mhealth/classification-digital-health-interventions/en/

[52] Anderson K, Burford O, Emmerton LL, et al.Mobile health apps to facilitate self-care: A qualitative study of user experiences. van Ooijen PMA, editor. PLoS One 2016;**11**:e0156164

[53] Wu Y, Yao X, Vespasiani G, et al. Mobile app-based interventions to support diabetes self-management: A systematic review of randomized controlled trials to identify functions associated with glycemic efficacy. JMIR mHealth and uHealth. 2017;**5**:e35

[54] Kitsiou S, Paré G, Jaana M, et al. Effectiveness of mHealth interventions for patients with diabetes: An overview of systematic reviews. Li D, editor. PLOS ONE. 2017;**12**:e0173160

[55] Free C, Phillips G, Felix L, et al. The effectiveness of M-health technologies for improving health and health services: A systematic review protocol. BMC Research Notes. 2010;**3**:250

[56] Woods KF, Johnson JA, Kutlar A, et al. Sickle cell disease telemedicine network for rural outreach. Journal of Telemedicine and Telecare. 2000;**6**:285-290

[57] Betjeman TJ, Soghoian SE, Foran MP. mHealth in Sub-Saharan Africa. International Journal of Telemedicine and Applications. 2013;**2013**:482324

[58] Bediang G, Perrin C, Ruiz de Castañeda R, et al. The RAFT telemedicine network: Lessons learnt and perspectives from a decade of educational and clinical services in low- and middle-incomes countries. Frontiers in Public Health. 2014;**2**:180

[59] Kruse CS, Goswamy R, Raval Y, et al. Challenges and opportunities of big data in health care: A systematic review. JMIR Medical Informatics. 2016;**4**:e38

[60] Suciu G, Suciu V, Martian A, et al. Big data, internet of things and cloud convergence—An architecture for secure E-health applications. Journal of Medical Systems. 2015;**39**:141

[61] Murray E, Hekler EB, Andersson G, et al. Evaluating digital health interventions: Key questions and approaches. American Journal of Preventive Medicine. 2016;**51**:843-851

[62] Vaghefi I, Tulu B. The continued use of mobile health apps: Insights from a longitudinal study. JMIR Mhealth Uhealth. 2019:7

[63] Robbins R, Krebs P, Jagannathan R, et al. Health app use among US mobile phone users: Analysis of trends by chronic disease status. JMIR mHealth and uHealth. 2017;**5**(12):e197

[64] Klein SK, McCarthy DM, Hostetter MH. Taking Digital Health to the Next Level: Promoting Technologies That Empower Consumers and Drive Health System Transformation. New York, NY United States: Commonwealth Fund; 2014

[65] Brahmbhatt R, Niakan S, Saha N, et al. Diabetes mHealth apps:

Designing for greater uptake. Studies in Health Technology and Informatics. 2017;**234**:49-53

[66] Senft N, Everson J. eHealth engagement as a response to negative healthcare experiences: Cross-sectional survey analysis. Journal of Medical Internet Research. 2018;**20**:e11034

[67] Lee AV, Moriarty JP, Borgstrom C, et al. What can we learn from patient dissatisfaction? Analysis of dissatisfying events at an academic medical center. Journal of Hospital Medicine. 2010;**5**:514-520

[68] Ward R, Taha KM. Patient Involvement as Experts in the Development and Assessment of a Smartphone App as a Patient Education Tool for the Management of Thalassemia and Iron Overload Syndromes. 2016; Available from: http://www.tandfonline.com/action/journalInformation?journalCode=ihem20. 10.1080/03630269.2016.1217875

[69] Burton C, Rycroft-Malone J. An untapped resource: Patient and public involvement in implementation. International Journal of Health Policy and Management. 2015;**4**:845-847

[70] Tatara N, Arsand E, Bratteteig T, et al. Usage and perceptions of a mobile self-management application for people with type 2 diabetes: Qualitative study of a five-month trial. Studies in Health Technology and Informatics. 2013;**192**:127-131

[71] Badawy SM, Cronin RM, Hankins J, et al. Patient-centered ehealth interventions for children, adolescents, and adults with sickle cell disease: Systematic review. Journal of Medical Internet Research. 2018;**20**:e10940

[72] Jacob SA, Carroll AE, Bennett WE. A feasibility study of telemedicine for paediatric sickle cell patients living in a rural medically underserved area. Journal of Telemedicine and Telecare. 2021;**27**:431-435

[73] Mgbako O, Miller EH, Santoro AF, et al. COVID-19, Telemedicine, and Patient Empowerment in HIV Care and Research. AIDS and Behavior. 2020;**24**:1990-1993

[74] Faezipour M, Abuzneid A. Smartphone-based self-testing of COVID- 19 using breathing sounds. Telemedicine and e-Health. 2020 Oct 1;**26**(10):1202-1205. DOI: 10.1089/TMJ.2020.0114

[75] DigitalHealth.net. Mobile health apps news in brief. Digital Health. 2021. Available from: https://www.digitalhealth.net/2021/01/mobile-health-apps-news-in-brief-7/ [Accessed: June 8, 2021]

[76] Faiz Aiman Bin Azhar1 JSD. A Systematic Review of Factors Influencing the Effective Use of mHealth Apps for Self-care. 2016 3rd International Conference On Computer And Information Sciences (ICCOINS). 2016. Available from: http://ieeexplore.ieee.org/stamp/stamp.jsp?arnumber=7783213.

[77] Krokstad S, Ding D, Grunseit AC, et al. Multiple lifestyle behaviours and mortality, findings from a large population-based Norwegian cohort study—The HUNT Study. BMC Public Health. 2017;**17**:58

[78] Cheng C, Brown RC, Cohen LL, et al. iACT—An interactive mHealth monitoring system to enhance psychotherapy for adolescents with sickle cell disease. Conference Proceedings. Annual International Conference of the IEEE Engineering in Medicine and Biology Society IEEE Engineering in Medicine and Biology Society Annual Conference. 2013;**2013**:2279-2282

[79] Badawy SM, Abebe KZ, Reichman CA, et al. Comparing the effectiveness of education versus digital cognitive behavioral therapy for adults with sickle cell disease: Protocol for the cognitive behavioral therapy and real-time pain management intervention for sickle cell via mobile applications (CaRISMA) Study. JMIR Reserach Protocol. 2021;**10**:e29014

[80] Kumar D, Arya M. mHealth is an innovative approach to address health literacy and improve patient-physician communication—An HIV testing exemplar. Journal of Mobile Technology in Medicine. 2015;**4**:25-30

[81] Parmanto B, Pramana G, Yu DX, et al. iMHere: A novel mHealth system for supporting self-care in management of complex and chronic conditions. JMIR mhealth and uhealth. 2013;**1**:e10

[82] Hou C, Xu Q, Diao S, et al. Mobile phone applications and self-management of diabetes: A systematic review with meta-analysis, meta-regression of 21 randomized trials and GRADE. Diabetes, Obesity and Metabolism. 2018. DOI: 10.1111/dom.13307

[83] Badawy SM, Cronin RM, Liem RI, et al. Digital behavioural interventions for people with sickle cell disease. The Cochrane Library. 2021;**2021**(4)

[84] Alberts NM, Badawy SM, Hodges J, et al. Development of the incharge health mobile app to improve adherence to hydroxyurea in patients with sickle cell disease: User-centered design approach. JMIR mHealth and uHealth. 2020;**8**(5):e14884

[85] Badawy SM. iManage: A novel self-management app for sickle cell disease. Pediatric Blood & Cancer. 2017;**64**:e26289

[86] Phillips S, Kanter J, Mueller M, et al. Feasibility of an mHealth self-management intervention for children and adolescents with sickle cell disease and their families. Translational Behavioral Medicine. 2021;**11**:724-732

[87] Issom D-Z, Hardy-Dessources M-D, Romana M, et al. Toward a conversational agent to support the self-management of adults and young adults with sickle cell disease: Usability and usefulness study. Front Digit Health. 2021 [cited 2021 May 22];**3**. DOI: 10.3389/fdgth.2021.600333/full

[88] Issom D-Z, Henriksen A, Woldaregay AZ, et al. Factors influencing motivation and engagement in mobile health among patients with sickle cell disease in low-prevalence, high-income countries: Qualitative exploration of patient requirements. JMIR Human Factors. 2020;**7**:e14599

[89] Michie S, van Stralen MM, West R. The behaviour change wheel: A new method for characterising and designing behaviour change interventions. Implementation Science. 2011;**6**:42

[90] Carey PJ. Addressing the global health burden of sickle cell disease. International Health. 2014

[91] Kulandaivelu Y, Lalloo C, Ward R, et al. Exploring the needs of adolescents with sickle cell disease to inform a digital self-management and transitional care program: Qualitative study. JMIR Pediatrics and Parenting. 2018;**1**:e11058

[92] Kumar R, Das A. The potential of mHealth as a game changer for the management of sickle cell disease in india. JMIR mHealth and uHealth. 2021;**9**:e25496

[93] Palermo TM, Zempsky WT, Dampier CD, et al. iCanCope with sickle cell pain: Design of a randomized

controlled trial of a smartphone and web-based pain self-management program for youth with sickle cell disease. Contemporary Clinical Trials. 2018;**74**:88-96

[94] Frost JR, Cherry RK, Faro EZ, et al. Improving sickle cell transitions of care through health information technology. American Journal of Preventive Medicine. 2016;**51**:S17-S23

[95] Johnson A, Yang F, Gollarahalli S, et al. Use of mobile health apps and wearable technology to assess changes and predict pain during treatment of acute pain in sickle cell disease: Feasibility study. JMIR mHealth and uHealth. 2019;7:e13671

[96] Ajayi TA, Salongo L, Zang Y, et al. Mobile health-collected biophysical markers in children with serious illness-related pain. Journal of Palliative Medicine. 2021;**24**:580-588

[97] Hankins JS, Shah N. Tackling adherence in sickle cell disease with mHealth. The Lancet Haematology. 2020;7:e713-e714

[98] Luo L, King AA, Carroll Y, et al. Electronic Health Record-Embedded Individualized pain plans for emergency department treatment of vaso-occlusive episodes in adults with sickle cell disease: Protocol for a preimplementation and postimplementation study. JMIR Res Protoc. 2021;**10**:e24818

[99] Veludhandi A, Ross D, Sinha CB, et al. A decision support tool for allogeneic hematopoietic stem cell transplantation for children with sickle cell disease: Acceptability and usability study. JMIR Formative Research. 2021;5:e30093

[100] Breslauer DN, Maamari RN, Switz NA, et al. Mobile phone based clinical microscopy for global health applications. PLoS One. 2009;**4**:e6320

[101] Barrett AN, McDonnell TCR, Chan KCA, et al. Digital PCR analysis of maternal plasma for noninvasive detection of sickle cell anemia. Clinical Chemistry. 2012;**58**:1026-1032

[102] WHO. WHO | Big data in global health: Improving health in low- and middle-income countries[Internet]. WHO. World Health Organization; [cited 2021 Jun 4]. Available from: https://www.who.int/bulletin/volumes/93/3/14-139022/en/

[103] Hafen E. Personal data cooperatives—A new data governance framework for data donations and precision health. In: Krutzinna J, Floridi L, editors. The Ethics of Medical Data Donation. Cham: Springer International Publishing; 2019. pp. 141-149. DOI: 10.1007/978-3-030-04363-6_9

[104] Odame I. Perspective: We need a global solution. Nature. 2014;**515**:S10

[105] Albers DJ, Levine M, Gluckman B, et al.Personalized glucose forecasting for type 2 diabetes using data assimilation. Mac Gabhann F, editor. PLOS Computational Biology. 2017;**13**:e1005232

[106] Information and Communication Technology for Development (ICT4D) [Internet]. Routledge and CRC Press. 2021. Available from: https://www.routledge.com/Information-and-Communication-Technology-for-Development-ICT4D/Heeks/p/book/9781138101814

[107] Azzopardi-Muscat N, Sørensen K. Towards an equitable digital public health era: Promoting equity through a health literacy perspective. European Journal of Public Health. 2019;**29**:13-17

[108] Kruse C, Betancourt J, Ortiz S, et al. Barriers to the use of mobile health in

improving health outcomes in developing countries: Systematic review. Journal of Medical Internet Research. 2019 Oct 9 [cited 2021 May 24];**21**(10). Available from: https://www.ncbi.nlm.nih.gov/pmc/articles/PMC6811771/

[109] Peng W, Kanthawala S, Yuan S, et al. A qualitative study of user perceptions of mobile health apps. BMC Public Health. 2016;**16**:1158

[110] Pratap A, Neto EC, Snyder P, et al. Indicators of retention in remote digital health studies: A cross-study evaluation of 100,000 participants. NPJ Digital Medicine. 2020;**3**:1-10

[111] Owen JE, Jaworski BK, Kuhn E, et al. mHealth in the Wild: Using Novel Data to Examine the Reach, Use, and Impact of PTSD Coach. JMIR Mental Health. 2015;**2**:e3935

[112] Baumel A, Muench F, Edan S, et al. Objective user engagement with mental health apps: Systematic search and panel-based usage analysis. Journal of Medical Internet Research. 2019;**21**:e14567

[113] Niazkhani Z, Toni E, Cheshmekaboodi M, et al. Barriers to patient, provider, and caregiver adoption and use of electronic personal health records in chronic care: A systematic review. BMC Medical Informatics and Decision Making. 2020;**20**:153

[114] Huang H-Y, Bashir M. Users' adoption of mental health apps: Examining the impact of information cues. JMIR mHealth and uHealth. 2017;**5**:e83

[115] Maiga G, Namagembe F. Predicting adoption of mHealth technology in resource constrained environments. In: IST-Africa Conference Proceedings. Vol. 2014. IEEE; 2014. pp. 1-12. Available from: http://ieeexplore.ieee.org/document/6880628/

[116] Vishwanath A, Scamurra SD. Barriers to the adoption of electronic health records: Using concept mapping to develop a comprehensive empirical model. Health Informatics Journal. 2007;**13**:119-134

[117] Hoque R, Sorwar G. Understanding factors influencing the adoption of mHealth by the elderly: An extension of the UTAUT model. International Journal of Medical Informatics. 2017;**101**:75-84

[118] Gagnon M-P, Ngangue P, Payne-Gagnon J, et al. m-Health adoption by healthcare professionals: A systematic review. Journal of the American Medical Informatics Association. 2016;**23**:212-220

[119] Adu MD, Malabu UH, Malau-Aduli AEO, et al. Users' preferences and design recommendations to promote engagements with mobile apps for diabetes self-management: Multi-national perspectives. PLoS One. [Internet]. 2018;**13**(12). [cited 2020 Jul 29]. Available from: https://www.ncbi.nlm.nih.gov/pmc/articles/PMC6287843/

[120] Birnbaum F, Lewis DM, Rosen R, et al. Patient engagement and the design of digital health. Academic Emergency Medicine. 2015;**22**:754-756

[121] Irizarry T, DeVito DA, Curran CR. Patient portals and patient engagement: A state of the science review. Journal of Medical Internet Research. 2015;**17**:e148

[122] Klasnja P, Kendall L, Pratt W, et al. Long-term engagement with health-management technology: A dynamic process in diabetes. AMIA. Annual Symposium proceedings AMIA Symposium. 2015;**2015**:756-765

[123] Scherer EA, Ben-Zeev D, Li Z, et al. Analyzing mHealth engagement: Joint models for intensively collected user engagement data. JMIR mHealth and uHealth. 2017;**5**:e1

[124] Miller S, Ainsworth B, Yardley L, et al. A framework for analyzing and measuring usage and engagement data (AMUsED) in digital interventions: Viewpoint. Journal of Medical Internet Research. 2019;**21**:e10966

[125] Rossmann C, Riesmeyer C, Brew-Sam N, et al. Appropriation of mobile health for diabetes self-management: Lessons from two qualitative studies. JMIR Diabetes. [Internet]. 2019 Mar 29 [cited 2021 May 24];**4**(1). Available from: https://www.ncbi.nlm.nih.gov/pmc/articles/PMC6460309/

[126] Klonoff DC. Benefits and limitations of self-monitoring of blood glucose. Journal of Diabetes Science and Technology. 2007;**1**:130-132

[127] Ancker JS, Witteman HO, Hafeez B, et al. "You Get Reminded You're a Sick Person": Personal data tracking and patients with multiple chronic conditions. Journal of Medical Internet Research. 2015;**17**:e202

[128] Krebs P, Duncan DT. Health app use among US mobile phone owners: A national survey. JMIR mHealth and uHealth. 2015;**3**:e101

[129] Yang D, Xue G, Fang X, et al. Incentive mechanisms for crowdsensing: Crowdsourcing with smartphones. IEEE/ACM Transactions on Networking. 2016;**24**:1732-1744

[130] Estellés-Arolas E, González-Ladrón-de-Guevara F. Towards an integrated crowdsourcing definition. Journal of Information Science. 2012;**38**:189-200

[131] Litchman ML, Walker HR, Fitzgerald C, et al. Patient-driven diabetes technologies: Sentiment and personas of the #WeAreNotWaiting and #OpenAPS movements. Journal of Diabetes Science and Technology. 2020;**14**:990-999

[132] UnitedHealth group acquires PatientsLikeMe. MobiHealthNews. 2019 [cited 2021 Jun 11]. Available from: https://www.mobihealthnews.com/content/unitedhealth-group-acquires-patientslikeme

[133] Li Y, Liu C, Du N, et al. Extracting medical knowledge from crowdsourced question answering website. IEEE Transactions on Big Data. 2020;**6**:309-321

[134] European Commission. Communication on enabling the digital transformation of health and care in the Digital Single Market; empowering citizens and building a healthier society | Shaping Europe's digital future. 2021. Available from: https://digital-strategy.ec.europa.eu/en/library/communication-enabling-digital-transformation-health-and-care-digital-single-market-empowering

[135] McCorkell L, Assaf GS, Davis EH, et al. Patient-led research collaborative: Embedding patients in the Long COVID narrative. Pain Reports. [Internet]. 2021;**6**(1). [cited 2021 Jun 6]. Available from: https://www.ncbi.nlm.nih.gov/pmc/articles/PMC8112577/

[136] Demonaco H, Oliveira P, Torrance A, et al. When patients become innovators. In: Tiwari R, Buse S, editors. Managing Innovation in a Global and Digital World: Meeting Societal Challenges and Enhancing Competitiveness. Wiesbaden: Springer Fachmedien; 2020. pp. 121-129. DOI: 10.1007/978-3-658-27241-8_9

[137] Labrique AB, Wadhwani C, Williams KA, et al. Best practices in scaling digital health in low and middle

income countries. Globalization and Health. 2018;**14**:103

[138] Proctor E, Silmere H, Raghavan R, et al. Outcomes for implementation research: Conceptual distinctions, measurement challenges, and research agenda. Administration and Policy in Mental Health. 2011;**38**:65-76

[139] Proctor EK, Landsverk J, Aarons G, et al. Implementation research in mental health services: An emerging science with conceptual, methodological, and training challenges. Administration and Policy in Mental Health. 2009;**36**. DOI: 10.1007/s10488-008-0197-4

Chapter 3

Detection and Management of Cerebral Vasculopathy

Françoise Bernaudin and Suzanne Verlhac

Abstract

Cerebral vasculopathy in children with sickle cell anemia is responsible for strokes and silent cerebral infarcts and is the most debilitating complication providing motor sequelae and cognitive deficiency. However, the most important advance in pediatric management is the detection of children at a risk of stroke using transcranial Doppler with chronic transfusion applied in children detected at risk, which reduces the stroke risk from 11% to less than 2%. In this chapter, we will describe the place of Doppler, magnetic resonance imaging (MRI), and magnetic resonance angiography (MRA) with neck assessment and the place of different treatments, i.e., chronic transfusion, hydroxyurea, new drugs, and stem cell transplantation.

Keywords: sickle cell disease, sickle cell anemia, stroke, silent cerebral infarcts, transcranial Doppler, color Doppler ultrasound, cerebral magnetic resonance imaging (MRI), cerebral magnetic resonance angiography (MRA), neck MRA, hydroxycarbamide, chronic transfusion, hematopoietic stem cell transplantation

1. Introduction

Sickle cell disease is a group of inherited hemoglobinopathies. The most severe types are hemoglobin SS and hemoglobin Sβ0 thalassemia, which are referred to as sickle cell anemia (SCA). It is a systemic disease characterized by a chronic hemolytic anemia, vaso-occlusive events, and susceptibility to bacterial infections with a great variability of the clinical presentation. The cerebral complications are particularly severe as they are a common cause of disability, often at a young age. Imaging plays a central role in the screening, diagnosis, and treatment optimization of patients with SCA.

2. Physiopathology

Deoxygenated hemoglobin S forms polymers with other hemoglobin molecules producing rigid filaments that deform the red blood cell into a sickle shape. The properties of the red blood cells are modified, making them fragile with a shortened life span, explaining the chronic hemolytic anemia, but also making them rigid, poorly deformable, and adherent to vascular endothelium. This causes intravascular sludging in terminal arterioles and capillaries and damage to the wall of large and medium arteries due to a cascade of endothelium activation, overexpression of adhesion molecules (endothelin 1 and BCAM), nitric oxide depletion, hypercoagulability, splitting of the internal elastic lamina, intimal hyperplasia, and smooth muscle proliferation that reduce the lumen diameter [1, 2]. The genesis of arterial lesions also involves arterial remodeling in response to high blood flow and velocities, disturbed wall shear stress associated with severe chronic anemia, and abnormalities of oxygen transport.

3. Cerebral manifestations

3.1 Overt ischemic stroke

3.1.1 Clinical symptoms and outcome

Ischemic stroke is a major cause of cognitive impairment, disability, and death. Strokes are suggested by hemiparesis, aphasia, dysphasia, or seizures and are frequently associated with vaso-occlusive crises and fever, although not always. Early on, survival is observed in 98% of children, with 62.5% of them exhibiting total motor recovery [3]. However, there are high risks of cognitive impairment and recurrence, which can reach 67% in the absence of transfusion, especially if there is an underlying arteriopathy [4]. SCA confers a higher risk of stroke in children than any other pediatric disease. Without prevention strategies, 11% of patients with SCA will suffer an overt stroke by the age of 20 years and 24% by the age of 45 years [3]. The risk of a first stroke is highest in the first decade of life, with a peak between the ages of 2 and 5 years.

3.1.2 Imaging

Acute infarction usually involves the parenchyma supplied by the carotid circulation, either in the territory of the middle cerebral artery (MCA) and/or anterior cerebral artery (ACA) or in the superficial and deep border zones between the anterior and MCA territories. It is related either to an arterial occlusion or to an acute drop of blood supply to the brain distal to an arterial stenosis.

Magnetic resonance imaging (MRI) is the preferred imaging modality because it shows the cytotoxic edema characteristic of ischemic stroke within the first hour of symptomatology, in contrast to brain computed tomography (CT), which is often normal during the first 24 hours. Within approximately 7 days of the onset of ischemia, the infarct will show high signal on diffusion weighted imaging (DWI) and low values on the apparent diffusion coefficient (ADC) map. The absence of high signal on fluid-attenuated inversion recovery (FLAIR) images indicates an infarct onset of less than 4–6 hours.

Time-of-flight magnetic resonance angiography (TOF MRA) of the Willis circle and of the cervical arteries shows an intra- and/or extracranial steno-occlusive arteriopathy in about three quarters of cases, most often of the anterior cerebral circulation.

3.1.3 Risk factors for ischemic stroke

The risk factors reported for overt ischemic strokes are a low baseline hemoglobin level, the rate of acute chest syndrome (ACS), a recent episode of ACS, and elevated systolic blood pressure [3]. Strokes can be promoted by hyperviscosity induced by transfusion of large volumes or by serere anemia during exchange in patients with stenosis. Cerebral desaturation is common in SCA patients, is correlated with the severity of anemia, and is a risk factor for stroke. Cerebral tissue hemoglobin saturation is positively correlated with hemoglobin, whereas cerebral blood flow (CBF) is negatively correlated with hemoglobin. Thus, in patients with severe anemia, there is a compensatory cerebral hyperperfusion in response to SCA-associated reduction in O_2-binding capacity. Cerebrovascular reserve capacities are already close to the maximum in SCA; thus, any decrease in CBF as observed during infection, fever, or ACS carries a risk of imbalance between brain oxygen demand and supply.

3.1.4 Prevention of recurrence

After a stroke, chronic transfusion to maintain the HbS level lower than 30% and hemoglobin between 9 and 11 g/dL has allowed reduction of the risk of recurrence from 67% to 10–20% [5, 6]. However, if chronic transfusion is stopped, the risk of recurrence is still about 50% [7]. Hydroxyurea has been used in patients with stroke history, but 19% recurrence was observed within 4 months [8]. Thereafter, a randomized trial comparing stroke recurrence on chronic transfusion + oral chelation to hydroxyurea + phlebotomies was prematurely stopped because of a significant higher incidence of recurrence in the hydroxyurea arm (7/67 versus 0/66 on chronic transfusion) [9]. Thus, chronic transfusion with oral chelation remains the reference treatment for secondary stroke prevention. In a review of a worldwide experience including 73 patients with a stroke history who have received a matched sibling donor stem cell transplantation (MSD-SCT), the occurrence of four hemorrhagic strokes (5.5%) has been reported, but no ischemic stroke recurrence [10, 11]. Thus, MSD-SCT offers the best prevention for secondary stroke. Different procedures of direct or indirect cerebral revascularization surgery in addition to regular blood transfusion have been proposed for patients with SCD, moyamoya syndrome, and a history of stroke or transient ischemic attack (TIA). However, the risk/benefit ratio of surgery in addition to other therapies, such as HSCT, is unclear, and prospective studies are needed.

3.2 Other acute neurovascular complications: Aneurysms, intracranial bleeding, fat embolism, posterior reversible encephalopathy syndrome (PRES), and reversible cerebral vasoconstriction syndrome (RCVS)

Aneurysm rupture is rarely responsible of intracranial hemorrhage in SCD pediatric patients, unlike in adults. However, saccular aneurysms are found on routine imaging in approximately 4% of children [12]. Compared to the general population, SCD patients are more likely to have multiple aneurysms. The internal carotid artery (ICA) is the most commonly involved artery followed by the posterior cerebral artery (PCA). Sustained endothelial injury causing vessel wall weakening is the presumed reason for the increased prevalence of aneurysms in patients with SCD.

Subarachnoid and intracerebral hemorrhage also occurs as a result of rupture of fragile moyamoya vessels or of venous sinus thrombosis, often in association with vaso-occlusive crisis, transfusion, or acute respiratory illness.

Fat embolism syndrome due to extensive bone marrow necrosis is a rare and devastating complication in sickle cell disease. Paradoxically, it affects exclusively patients with mild forms of SCD, predominantly HbSC and HbSβ^+. A significant number of cases occur in the context of human parvovirus B19 infection. The diagnosis is made by cerebral MRI showing innumerable bilateral punctate foci of restricted diffusion on diffusion-weighted imaging in a starfield pattern throughout the brain and associated petechial hemorrhage on susceptibility-weighted imaging. Early recognition and intervention with red cell exchange transfusion can be life-saving [13].

Posterior reversible encephalopathy syndrome (PRES) has been reported in the context of hypertension and cyclosporine use for nephrotic syndrome, as well as after ACS.

Reversible cerebral vasoconstriction syndrome (RCVS) has been reported in children with SCD. Arterial constriction affects not only large but also distal arteries of both anterior and posterior circulations and is rapidly reversible. RCVS can be complicated by cerebral infarction, bleeding, or PRES.

4. Transcranial and neck Doppler ultrasound (Doppler-US), an essential tool in the management of sickle cell anemia

4.1 Rationale

Transcranial and neck Doppler ultrasound (Doppler-US) is a noninvasive technique, which measures flow velocities in the large cerebral arteries and can determine the risk of stroke in children with SCA [14]. A risk of stroke of 10% per year was found in SCA children with a mean velocity in the terminal ICA or MCA ≥200 cm/s versus 2% if velocities were normal [15]. In the Stroke Prevention in Sickle Cell Anemia (STOP) trial [16], the risk of stroke among children with high transcranial Doppler (TCD) velocities was reduced by 90% by maintaining HbS concentrations at <30% through chronic transfusion therapy. Doppler-US is also used to diagnose and monitor cerebral arteriopathy in an acute or steady state. Several cohort studies have shown the remarkable effectiveness of chronic transfusion, including the French study that found a reduction in the risk of stroke at age 18 to 1.9%, compared with the historical risk of 11% [17].

4.2 Anatomy review of the cerebral arteries

The internal carotid artery is a terminal branch of the common carotid artery. It arises around the level of the fourth cervical vertebra. Terminologia Anatomica in 1998 subdivided the artery into four segments: “cervical,” “petrous,” “cavernous,” and “supraclinoid” (**Figure 1**).

The cervical segment runs vertically upward in the carotid sheath anteriorly and medially to the internal jugular vein in front of the transverse processes of the upper three cervical vertebrae and then enters the carotid canal of the temporal bone in the base of the skull. It does not give any branch.

The petrous segment runs from carotid canal to foramen lacerum within the petrous temporal bone. It first has a vertical course and then a horizontal course along the middle ear.

The cavernous segment passes from the petrous apex to the dural ring of the anterior clinoid process surrounded by cavernous sinus where its course describes a hairpin bend, called the siphon.

DOI: http://dx.doi.org/10.5772/intechopen.105099

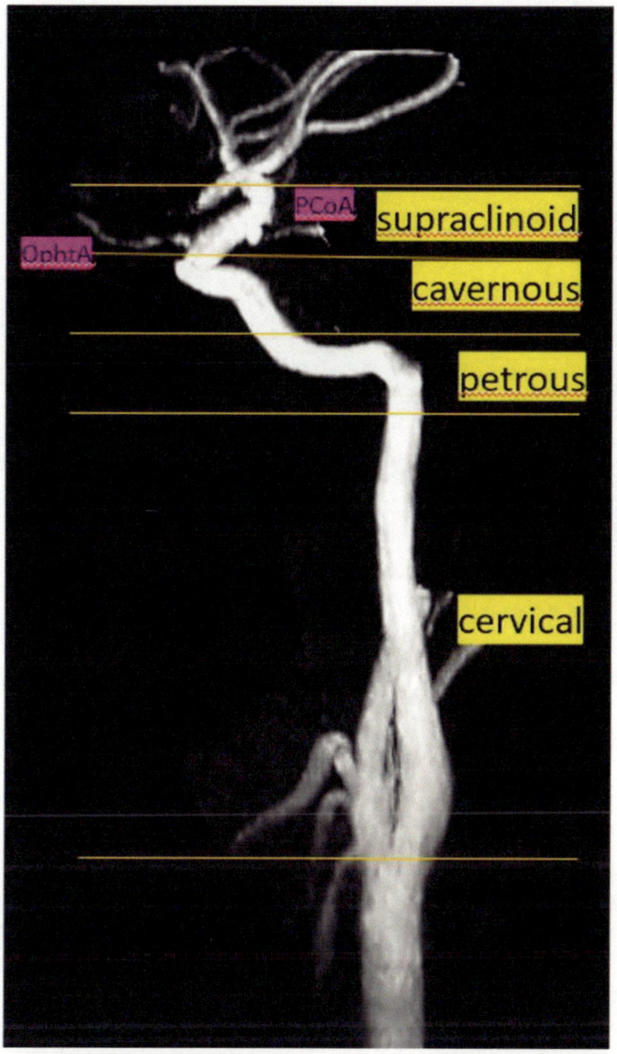

Figure 1.
The four segments of the internal carotid artery. Lateral view.

Then, *the supraclinoid segment*, also called cerebral segment, runs above the clinoid process through the dura into the subarachnoid space. Several important branches arise from the supraclinoid carotid, such as ophthalmic, posterior communicating, and anterior choroidal arteries. It gives two terminal branches: the MCA and ACA.

The circle of Willis is an anastomotic arterial ring located at the base of the brain that communicates blood flow between the two hemispheres and between the anterior and posterior arterial circulations. It is formed by the initial segment of the ACAs, the anterior communicating artery, the two posterior communicating arteries, the two ICAs, and the initial segment of the two posterior cerebral arteries (**Figure 2**). These shunts are involved in the case of occlusion or severe stenosis of a segment. Variations are possible in the A1, P1, and posterior communicating segments, but they are rare in pediatric age.

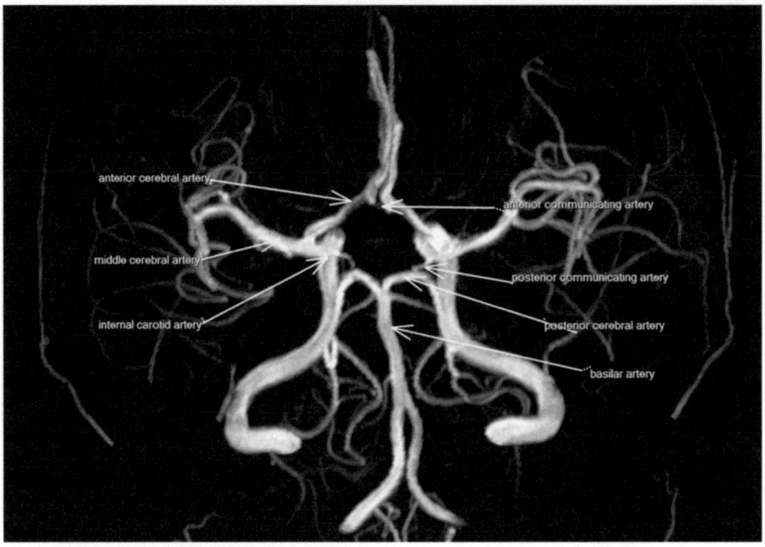

Figure 2.
3D TOF MRA. Axial view of the circle of Willis.

The most important branch of the ICA in diameter and length is the *MCA*, which supplies most of the lateral aspect of the hemisphere and provides 60–80% of the hemisphere's blood flow. After its origin, the MCA runs laterally and horizontally toward the Sylvian fissure. Its terminal branches anastomose with the terminal branches of the anterior and posterior cerebral arteries at the surface of the brain.

The *ACA* is the other terminal branch of the ICA. It has a horizontal course anteriorly and medially in its precommunicating A1 segment. At the entrance to the interhemispheric fissure, it anastomoses with the contralateral ACA via the anterior communicating artery, which participates in the circle of Willis. Downstream of the communicating artery, the ACA curves upward and runs parallel to the contralateral artery in the hemispheric fissure.

The *basilar artery* has a vertical ascending course on the anterior surface of the pons in the basilar sulcus. At the level of the peduncles, it gives the two posterior cerebral arteries.

4.3 Transcranial and neck Doppler ultrasound methodology

4.3.1 Equipment and acoustic window

Historically, validation data used a nonimaging dedicated TCD technique by probing the temporal acoustic windows to determine flow velocities in the terminal ICA and proximal MCA. Arteries are identified by the depth of the sample volume, the direction of blood flow relative to the probe, and the position and angulation of the probe relative to the patient' head. In contrast, the TCD imaging technique combines pulsed-wave Doppler ultrasound with a color-coded cross-sectional view of the intonation area to visualize the arteries. Today, all centers in France and more than half in the United States and Great Britain use a color Doppler ultrasound device, which is routinely used in imaging and vascular medicine units.

Familiarity with the technique and ease of use, combined with a quicker achievement of competencies, favor this technique, and this is the one we describe here. The probe is either a sector or phased array cardiac or dedicated probe with a small imaging footprint and a Doppler frequency of 1.8 or 2 MHz to adequately penetrate through the skull. Transcranial and cervical Doppler ultrasound allows a real-time assessment of cerebral arterial hemodynamic. The objective is to assess the circulatory velocities of the large intracranial arteries and the cervical segment of the ICAs to detect abnormal velocities. The probe is positioned on specific sites, called acoustic windows, which are two temporal windows on the right and left temporal bones, the suboccipital and two submandibular windows under the mandible. The scan bilaterally records the MCA, ACA, PCA and the supraclinoid and cavernous segments of the ICA and to finish the complete course of the cervical extracranial segment of the ICA (eICA). The basilar artery is assessed by the suboccipital approach, placing the probe at the tip of the neck, just below the hairline, and angling it superiorly. It looks like a Y encoded in blue as the blood flow is going away from the transducer.

4.3.2 Settings

The settings must be adapted to the age and pathology of the patients, who have chronic anemia. The field of exploration will be of 8–10 cm, the velocity scale of the color Doppler from −100 to +100 cm/s, as well as that of the pulsed Doppler, which has to be increased in case of spectral aliasing. The pulsed Doppler gate should be wide enough (4–5 mm) to capture all the velocities within the vessel lumen, the fastest flows having a lower intensity. The size of the spectrum display and the gain should be adapted to allow an optimal tracing of the velocity spectrum.

4.3.3 Procedure of the examination

The examination is performed with the patient in the supine position and the examiner siting bedside on the patient's right, as for an abdominal scan, with the forearm resting on the patient's shoulder or chest to assure good stability and a little restraint of the child (**Figure 3**).

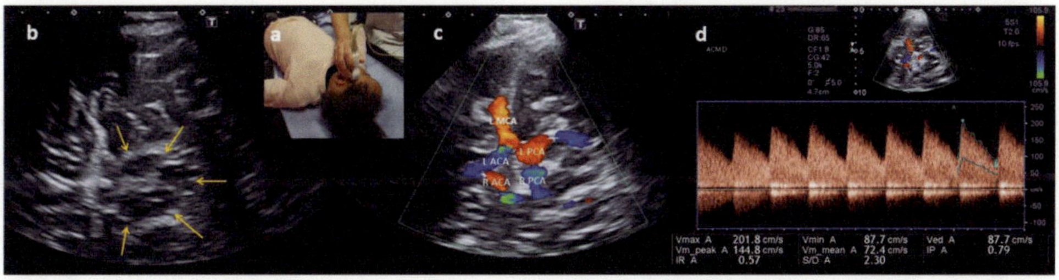

Figure 3.
Temporal window. (a) Positioning of the probe on the patient's temple. (b) Identification of the hypoechoic butterfly-shaped mesencephalic brainstem in a gray-scale axial view of the brain base. (c) In the color mode, the circle of Willis projects forward. (d) Spectral display of MCA velocities. Normal time average mean of maximal velocity (TAMV) 144 cm/s.

4.3.3.1 Temporal window

The probe is placed in front of the upper part of the tragus of the ear and above the zygoma, and an axial gray-scale view of the base of the brain is obtained depicting the hypoechoic, butterfly-shaped mesencephalic brainstem, surrounded by hyperechoic subarachnoid cisterns, which is the reference landmark. In the color mode, the circle of Willis projects anteriorly. The MCA, which is the main artery receiving 75–80% of the ICA flow, courses laterally toward the probe from the ICA bifurcation and is encoded in red. After switching to the spectral Doppler mode, the Doppler sample gate is placed on the ICA bifurcation and moved toward the periphery along the MCA. Since the objective of the examination is to detect focal acceleration of blood flow, it is important to carefully explore the entire course of the artery by sweeping the sample gate along the MCA and the ICA during spectral recording and by optimizing the recording at each depth by tilting and sliding the transducer slightly in order to get the highest velocity. Expert operators rely on the sound signal: the higher the pitch, the higher the velocity. Blood flow spectrum is above baseline. Two to three velocity recordings are captured from ICA bifurcation toward the periphery, and the highest velocity is collected. By moving the Doppler gate deeper, the proximal segment of the ACA is then examined, which is coded blue as the blood flow moves toward the midline away from the probe. After angling the probe inferiorly, the ICA is visualized as two round structures, because it is seen in transverse section as ICA has a vertical course. The red structure is the supraclinoid segment, and the blue structure, which is slightly inferior and anterior, is the cavernous hairpin segment. To obtain a good view, the transducer often needs to be slid posteriorly. Next, the PCA is scanned and coded red in the proximal segment and blue as it travels around the cerebral peduncle. After completing the study on one side, it is repeated on the other side after asking the child to turn his head to the other side.

4.3.3.2 Suboccipital window

Terminal segments of the vertebral arteries and basilar artery can be visualized via the suboccipital window with the patient in the lateral decubitus. The probe is placed in the middle position at the top of the neck right below the hairline and angled superiorly. The Y-shaped, blue-encoded confluence of the vertebral and basilar arteries is depicted in an oblique frontal view.

4.3.3.3 Submandibular window

The probe is placed under the angle of the mandible, directed upward, parallel to the midline. The extracranial cervical segment of the ICA (eICA) is visualized in a frontal view, encoded in blue, medial to the internal jugular vein encoded in red. The course of the artery is studied, which can be straight or sinuous, and possible blood flow acceleration zones are detected by the presence of aliasing. The spectral display of velocities is acquired along the entire course of the artery, from origin to entry into the carotid canal, by moving the Doppler gate along the artery in search of focal acceleration of blood flow (**Figure 4**). It is important not to compress the artery with the probe, in order not to induce false positive.

4.3.3.4 Tips and tricks

No angle correction should be made because arteries are short and sinuous. Moreover, stroke risk has been stratified using dedicated TCD without angle

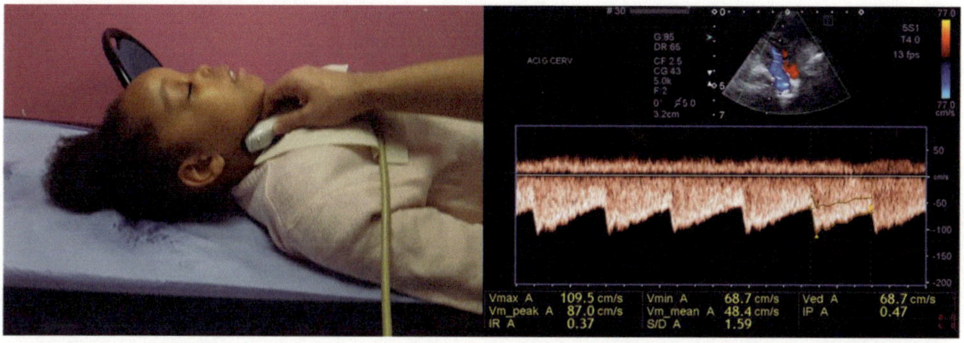

Figure 4.
Submandibular window. (a) Position of the probe. (b) Color mapping of the ICA and internal jugular vein and spectral display of velocities.

correction. Introducing an inappropriate angle correction would result in overestimation of flow velocities, potentially leading to overtreatment. It should be noted that an incorrect 60° angle correction will double the value of the measured velocity value and result in a very high risk of false diagnosis. The tracing is assumed to be obtained at an optimal angle of 0°.

4.3.3.5 Indication of the exam

Doppler-US screening is recommended for children with SCA from the second year of life. Children should then be rescanned annually if normal, quarterly if conditional, and chronic transfusion should be initiated in case of abnormal velocity. Doppler-US cannot be replaced by MRA, as it is a more sensitive technique and detects arterial disease at an earlier stage than MRA. However, children with abnormal velocity and stenosis on MRA are at higher risk for stroke than those with an abnormal Doppler alone. MRA is recommended in children with abnormal Doppler-US as well as in children with inadequate exam when there is no patent acoustic window.

The utility of using Doppler-US to monitor children with established stroke and cerebral vasculopathy is unclear. A multidisciplinary approach to decision is required.

4.3.4 Factors influencing velocities

4.3.4.1 Aging

Velocities increase during the first years of life, reaching a maximum value between the fourth and the sixth year of life, and decrease thereafter to about 70% of the maximal velocities by the age of 18 years.

Figure 5 shows the mean velocity [95% confidence interval (CI)] at annual check-up during aging in SCA children of the Créteil newborn cohort in right and left MCAs, ACAs, ICAs, and eICAs.

Velocities in the vertebrobasilar circulation are lower than in the carotid circulation.

4.3.4.2 Hematocrit

There is an inverse linear relationship between hematocrit and velocity. Velocities increase in anemia due to increased cardiac output, decreased blood viscosity, and

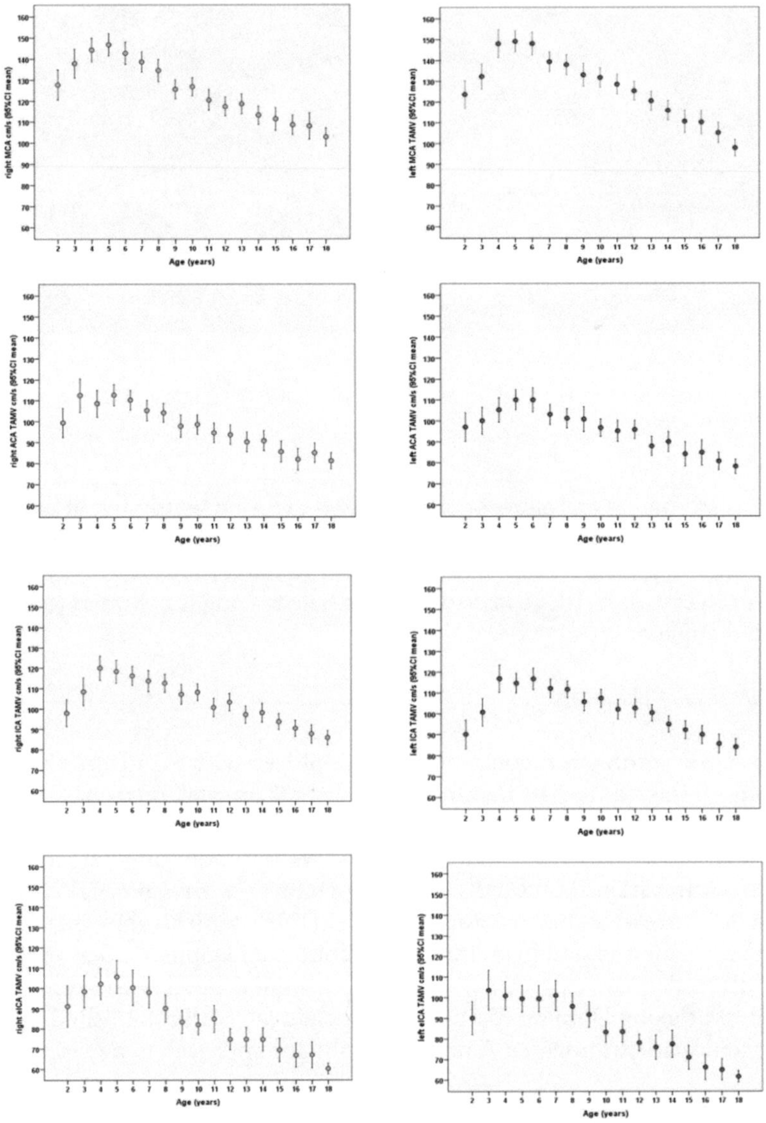

Figure 5.
Outcome of cerebral velocities during aging in SCA children.

decreased intracranial resistance, allowing a sustained normal oxygenation of the brain. This explains why children with SCA have high velocities, even in the absence of a stenosis. Consequently, thresholds for normal/abnormal velocities are different in SCA children, compared to non-SCA children.

4.3.4.3 Carbon dioxide (CO2)

Carbon dioxide (CO2) is a powerful modulator of CBF and intracranial velocities, as is the partial pressure of oxygen (PaO2). Hypercapnia induces vasodilatation, a dramatic increase in velocities, and a decrease in pulsatility index (PI) and resistance index (RI). In turn, hyperventilation, via a reduction of PaCO2 and hypocapnic alkalosis, induces the constriction of distal intracranial arterioles, a significant decrease in intracranial velocities, and an increase in PI and RI. These mechanisms called cerebral vasoreactivity are mediated via changes in extracellular pH. Sleep may increase velocities slightly due to hypercapnia. Crying may decrease velocities due to hypocapnia. Fever increases blood flow by about 10%. As a consequence, examination should be performed in a healthy condition, and children must remain awake during the exam. Sedation of young children is not recommended. The usual preparation and diversion techniques in pediatrics will be used (watching video, soft words from the attendant, etc.).

4.4 Detection of abnormally high cerebral velocities

4.4.1 Time average mean of maximal velocity (TAMV)

Three key parameters can be obtained from the Doppler spectrum display: flow direction, velocities, and indices for arterial resistances. Flow direction can be assessed by the color code. By convention, blood flow toward the transducer is encoded in red and is above baseline, and blood flow away from the transducer is encoded in blue and is under the baseline. The velocity parameter that is used in children with SCA is the time average mean of maximum velocity (TAMV), also called mean velocity, which can be measured by the manual or automated outlining of the envelope of the spectral display over one or a few cardiac cycles. Pay attention that TAMV is different from maximum systolic velocity. Doppler-US looks for abnormal blood flow acceleration signaling hemodynamic stenosis of the artery indicative of an increased risk of arteriopathy and stroke. Remember that as long as blood flow is maintained downstream of the stenosis, a reduction in luminal caliber is coupled with an acceleration of flow.

TAMV is used to classify the scan. Intracranial velocity thresholds for risk stratification are adapted from the STOP study [15]. If velocities in at least one intracranial artery are equal to or higher than 200 cm/s, the scan is abnormal indicating a 40% stroke risk within 36 months; between 170 and 199 cm/s, it is conditional with a 7% stroke risk; and it is normal if velocity in any artery is lower than 170 cm/s with a stroke risk of only 2%. For the cervical ICA, the abnormally high velocity threshold is 160 cm/s [18].

The absence of the visibility of MCA in a patient with a patent temporal window and a TAMV below 50 cm/s in the MCA are also abnormal findings and are associated with an increased risk of stroke. Note that low velocity is significant only in an MCA, whereas low velocity in the proximal segment of the ACA probably corresponds to the constitutional hypoplasia of the artery with low blood flow. Low MCA velocities are due to measurements within poststenotic main artery or within collaterals moya-like in the presence of an MCA occlusion or to re-entry flow in the MCA from a communicating artery in the presence of an occlusion of the homolateral ICA or in the presence of a large infarcted area with little metabolic demand and marked reduction of flow, all these suggesting the possibility of severe vasculopathy and the need for an MRI/MRA. Usually, MCA spectral display is demodulated with a resistance index IR < 0.45 and a pulsatility index IP < 0.60.

4.4.2 Incidence of abnormal cerebral arterial velocities

4.4.2.1 Abnormally high intracranial velocity (intracranial TAMV ≥200 cm/s)

In STOP-I, the classification at initial TCD examinations was: 67% normal, 17.6% conditional, 9.3% abnormal, and 6% inadequate. The follow-up of the Créteil SCD

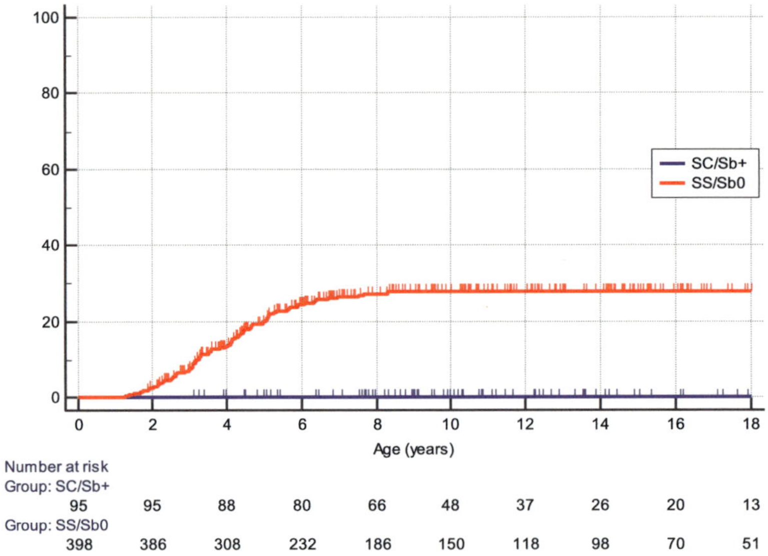

Figure 6.
Cumulative incidence of intracranial TAMV ≥200 cm/s in the Créteil newborn SCD cohort: 27.6% (95%CI: 22.8–32.4%) in SCA versus 0% in SC/Sb + children by 10 years of age (p < 0.001).

newborn cohort, assessed since 1992 by TCD as soon as 18 months of age, showed that abnormally high velocity occurred at median (range) age of 3.6 years (1.3–8.3 years) in SCA patients and was not observed in SC/Sb + patients, whereas the cumulative incidence of abnormally high velocity in the SS/Sb0 patients reached a plateau of about 30% by 9 years of age (**Figure 6**) [19].

4.4.2.2 Conditional velocity (intracranial TAMV 170–199 cm/s)

In the Créteil cohort, the rate of conversion from conditional to abnormal TCD was 34.5%. The median age of conditional TCD was 2.5 years (range, 1.2–5.5) and the median delay 1.1 years (range, 0.03–7). Age below 4 years old was a significant risk factor for conversion (odds ratio (OR) = 6.7; 95%CI: 1.7–27; $p = 0.007$) [17]. In the STOP study, the conversion risk was 97% in very young children with two consecutive conditional TCD examinations, and 13% in teenagers seen for the first time at the age of 14 years. This demonstrated the need for repeat screening of children with SCA throughout their childhood and argued for the closer monitoring of those with conditional TCD.

4.4.2.3 Abnormally high extracranial velocity (eICA TAMV ≥160 cm/s)

A cross-sectional study performed in two centers in France (Debré and Créteil) reported that eICA TAMV ≥160 cm/s was present in 9.2% of SCA patients without concomitant abnormal intracranial velocities and were strongly associated with eICA MRA-defined stenosis. Thus, this threshold was used to define abnormally high eICA velocities [18]. This study also showed that low hemoglobin level and tortuosities were associated risk factors.

The follow-up of the newborn Créteil cohort showed that abnormal high eICA TAMVs were detected at median (range) of 5.0 (1.3–10.0) years. The cumulative incidence of eICA TAMV ≥160 cm/s in SCA children was 17.4% by 10 years of age. The probability of developing high TAMV eICA ≥160 cm/s began in the second year of life, at the same age as intracranial velocities, and reached a plateau at age 10 years. Most often, eICA TAMV ≥160 cm/s was isolated (without intracranial TAMV ≥200 cm/s) and the probability of isolated eICA TAMV ≥160 cm/s was 13.8% by age 10 (**Figures** 7 and **8**) [19].

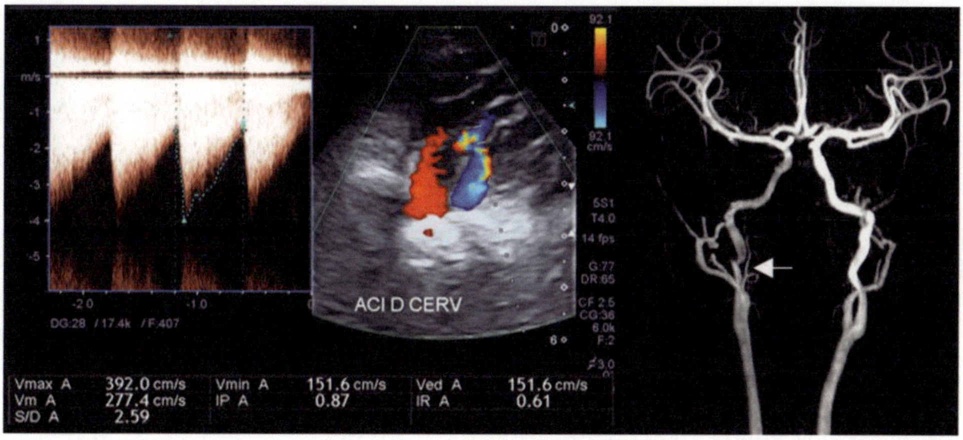

Figure 7.
Six-year-old boy without history of stroke. Routine Doppler ultrasound detected focal acceleration in the middle part of the right cervical ICA with TAMV 277 cm/s. 3D TOF MRA shows focal marked narrowing of the artery associated with a kink. Notice the hypointensity of the right ICA due to poor flow.

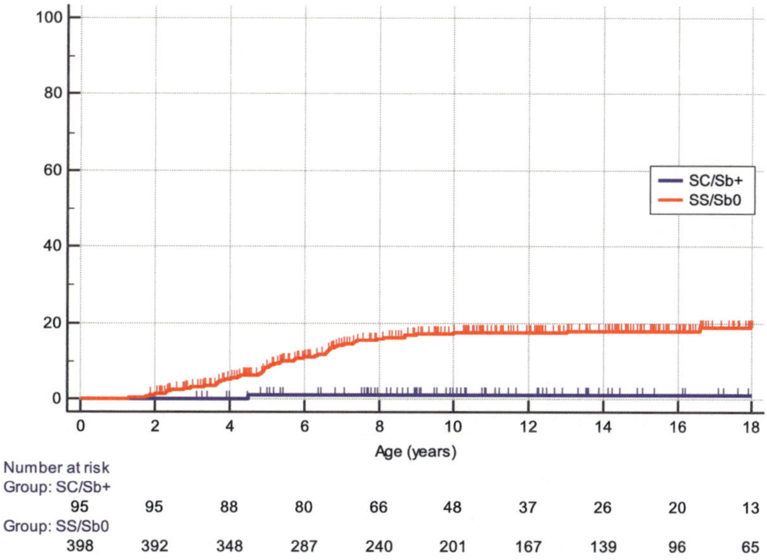

Figure 8.
Cumulative incidence of eICA TAMV ≥160 cm/s in the Créteil newborn SCD cohort: 17.4% (95%CI: 13.2–21.6%) in SCA versus 1.1% (95%CI: 0–3.4%), in SC/Sb + children ($p < 0.001$) by 10 years of age.

4.4.3 Predictors for abnormal velocities

Among genetic markers, G6PD deficiency and the absence of alpha-thalassemia have been described to be predictive risk factors for abnormal intracranial velocities [20]. Among biological parameters recorded during the second year of life away from vaso-occlusive crisis or transfusion and always before any intensive therapy, severe anemia, hyperleukocytosis, and hyperreticulocytosis were predictive risk factors for intracranial velocities.

For eICA velocities, the presence of tortuosities and severe anemia were risk factors for abnormal high eICA velocities [18].

4.5 Prevention of abnormally high cerebral velocities

4.5.1 Intracranial velocities

Hydroxyurea treatment in SCA children by inducing an increase of HbF% reduces the polymerization of HbS and hemolysis and decreases white blood cell (WBC) and reticulocyte counts [21]. The safety of its use in young children has been proven [22] (Baby-Hug) in high- and low-income countries such as in Africa [23, 24]. All these effects allow the reduction of cerebral velocities [25, 26], and several studies have shown the reduction of the incidence of abnormally high intracranial velocities, of conversion from conditional to abnormal velocities, and of strokes [27–33]. Similarly, in the Créteil newborn cohort, among the 53 children for whom HU was introduced before year 3, only 2/53 (3.8%) developed abnormal intracranial velocities, while the incidence after later HU initiation was 99/345 (28.7%), $p < 0.001$. Thus, we confirm that hydroxyurea significantly reduces the risk to develop abnormal intracranial velocities and could be systematically and early given as recommended by US guidelines [34].

4.5.2 Extracranial velocities

As we have shown that high eICA velocities were associated with severe anemia and presence of tortuosities themselves favored by anemia, drugs such hydroxyurea or voxelotor [35] could be good candidates to decrease eICA velocities.

4.6 Management of abnormally high cerebral velocities

4.6.1 Chronic transfusion

The STOP-1 trial randomizing chronic transfusion versus simple observation for 3 years in children with TAMV ≥200 cm/s in MCA or ICA demonstrated that stroke risk was highly significantly reduced by 92% with chronic transfusion ($p < 0.001$) [16]. Thereafter, the randomized STOP-2 trial posed the question of the required duration of chronic transfusion and compared pursuing to stopping chronic transfusion in patients who had been on chronic transfusion for at least 30 months, had normalized velocities on chronic transfusion, and had no severe stenosis. A high rate of stroke and abnormal TCD recurrence was observed after the discontinuation of chronic transfusion [36]. TCD screening and chronic transfusion applied in children detected at risk by TCD was the most significant progress in the managing of children with SCA reducing the risk of stroke by age 18 years from 11% [3] to less than 2% in the Créteil newborn cohort [17]. However, considering the risks related to long-term chronic transfusion, such as those of alloimmunization and iron overload and the benefits obtained with hydroxyurea by reducing hemolysis, hyperleukocytosis, and anemia severity, it seemed interesting to switch from chronic transfusion to HU patients who had normalized velocities on chronic transfusion and had no stenosis [37].

4.6.2 Switch to hydroxyurea

In the United States and Canada, a randomized, noninferiority trial comparing continued chronic transfusion versus hydroxyurea after at least 12 months of chronic transfusion has been conducted between 2011 and 2013 in patients with no severe vasculopathy [38]. Noninferiority was met, but the follow-up was short, with only 50% enrolled having reached the 2-year follow-up, the mean 4.5 years' duration of chronic transfusion prior to enrolment was long, and the mean age at enrolment was 9.7; therefore, most of patients might have not have been at risk at the time of enrolment [10].

In Créteil, France, all the SCA children with TAMV ≥200 cm/s patients were placed on long-term chronic transfusion, but those with normalized velocities on chronic transfusion and no stenosis were switched to hydroxyurea since 1998, with a quarterly control of TCD and immediate reinitiation of chronic transfusion in case of reversion to abnormal velocities [10]. No stroke was observed, but reversions occurred in about one-third of the patients, requiring chronic transfusion reinitiation [10]. Thus, longer follow-up periods are required to ensure that such early switch to hydroxyurea is safe.

4.6.3 Stem cell transplantation

The French multicenter prospective DREPAGREFFE trial compared outcomes after matched sibling donor stem cell hematopoietic transplantation (MSD-HSCT) versus chronic transfusion for at least 1 year in children with SCA and a history of abnormal cerebral velocities. This trial showed that transplantation compared to standard care was associated at 1 and 3 years with a significant reduction in cerebral velocities of 40 cm/s [39]. This large difference favoring the transplantation group confirms previous findings in a retrospective cohort study. The result is likely due in part to the correction of anemia, as well as to the exclusive presence of normal red cells after transplantation in contrast to the simultaneous presence of normal and sickle red cells in the circulation after transfusion.

4.6.4 Recommendations for the follow-up of cerebral velocities and management of abnormally high velocities

Recommendations in patients with SCA with abnormally high cerebral velocities have been recently updated in UK [40], United States [41], and Brazil [42]. We present here the protocol proposed in France for the follow-up and management in patients with abnormally high intracranial or cervical arterial velocities.

It is recommended to assess SCA children with intracranial and cervical Doppler ultrasound as soon as the second year of life, annually if intracranial TAMV <170 cm/s and eICA <140 cm/s, quarterly if conditional TCD (intracranial TAMV 170–199 cm</s or eICA 140–160 cm/s.

For children younger than 6 years with high conditional TCD (185–199 cm/s), we recommend to control TCD within a month.

For all children with intracranial or cervical TAMV ≥ 200 cm/s, it is important to analyze on the same day the blood parameters.

If Hb is <6 g/dL or < 20% baseline Hb level, as observed, for example, with acute splenic sequestration or parvoB19-related erythroblastopenia, we recommend to transfuse once time and to check TCD at 1 and 3 months post-transfusion.

If Hb is in the range of baseline Hb, we recommended to initiate monthly chronic transfusion with the goal to maintain Hb between 9 and 11 g/dL and HbS% lower than 30%. Exchange transfusions are more efficient to decrease HbS level and to avoid hyperviscosity and iron overload; however, they are more difficult to initiate in very young children (<1–4 years) and simple transfusions (10–15 mL/kg according to Hb level) are most often sufficient to maintain HbS lower than 30% after two transfusions. Cerebral MRI/MRA with neck MRA is performed after two or three transfusions. Images are better after the correction of severe anemia in order to discriminate anemia-related turbulences from true stenosis. Moreover, sedation required in very young children will be safer in transfused children.

Thereafter, the duration of chronic transfusion will depend on the presence or absence of stenosis on MRA and neck MRA, on the evolution of velocities, and on the age of the child.

For patients with MRA-depicted stenosis, we recommend to maintain chronic transfusion until stenosis disappearance or stem cell transplantation. At date, we do not know if there is a benefit to associate HU to chronic transfusion in these patients.

For patients without MRA-depicted stenosis, we recommend to initiate hydroxyurea treatment if not already given and to maintain chronic transfusion at least until the maximal tolerated dose of hydroxyurea is reached. US recommendations are to transfuse for at least 1 year. However, the suitable duration of chronic transfusion has not been clearly defined. We consider that the duration of chronic transfusion should be adapted to the age of the child and to velocities.

- For children with normalized TAMV (< 170 cm/s), chronic transfusion is stopped. For children younger than 6 years, it is safe to control TCD every 3 months until age 6. For those older than 6 years, annual TCD control is recommended.

- For children with conditional TAMV (170–199 cm/s), we recommend to maintain chronic transfusion until age 6. Thereafter, on hydroxyurea, high conditional TCD should be controlled every 3 months.

- Any reversion to abnormal TAMV (≥200 cm/s) requires to reinitiate chronic transfusion.

For all children with SCA, we recommend to perform cerebral MRI/MRA with neck MRA every 2 years for children older than 5 years or earlier in those already on chronic transfusion for abnormally high velocities.

Familial human leukocyte antigen (HLA) typing should be recommended in children with a history of abnormally high velocities. For children with an HLA-identical sibling donor, HSCT is recommended in all children having cerebral arterial stenosis and/or ischemic cerebral lesions or persistent abnormally high velocities or cognitive deficiency.

For eICA TAMV 160–199 cm/s, we recommend to perform MRI/MRA with neck MRA and to initiate chronic transfusion in presence of eICA-stenosis. In absence of eICA-stenosis, we recommend to initiate hydroxyurea if not already given.

5. Cerebral arterial stenoses

5.1 MRA-defined large vessel arteriopathy

TOF MRA has a good sensitivity and specificity for detecting steno-occlusive lesions in cerebral arteries (**Figure 9**) [43].

SCA arteriopathy is a progressive stenotic arteriopathy of the large cerebral arteries affecting the proximal MCAs, proximal ACAs, and ICAs in their intracranial but also cervical portions. They may be associated with the development of bypassing collateral vessels in the basal ganglia, known as moyamoya, from the Japanese expression describing the angiogram appearing like a "puff of smoke." Posterior pial collateral vessel circulation is not rare (**Figure 10**).

We showed in the Créteil newborn cohort that cervical ICA arteriopathy develops as soon as the second year of life, reaching a plateau at about 10 years of age, similarly to intracranial arteriopathy [19]. Extra and intracranial arteriopathies are most often not linked, and eICA assessment identifies 13.5% additional patients at a risk of stroke (eICA-TAMMV ≥200 cm/s or eICA stenosis) who have no intracranial arteriopathy. Cervical stenoses are frequently associated with severe tortuosities

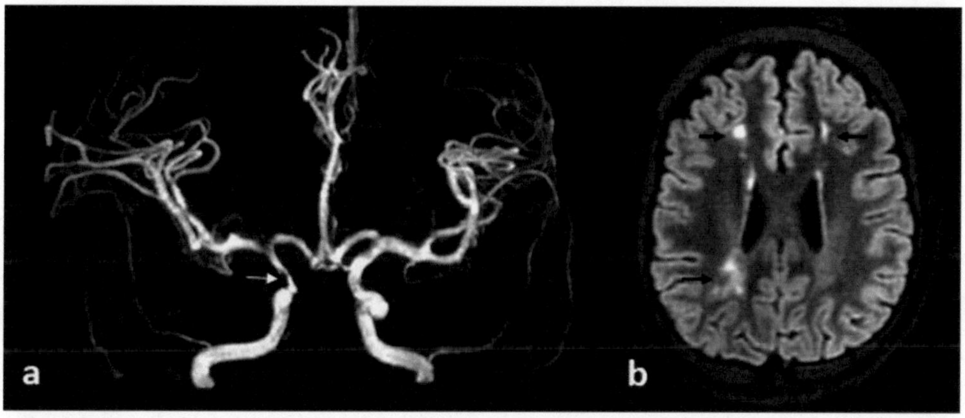

Figure 9.
3D TOF MRA. (a) Frontal view of the anterior circulation after segmentation. Marked narrowing of the supraclinoid segment of the right ICA, proximal right ACM, and right ACA. (b) Axial FLAIR image showing bilateral hyperintensities in the deep borderzones.

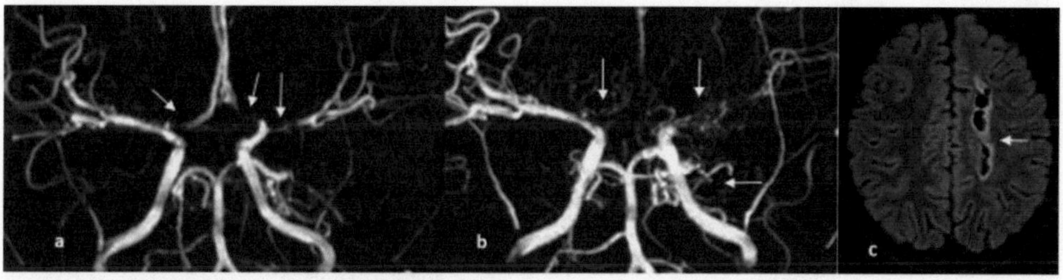

Figure 10.
SCA patient who suffered a stroke at the age of 3 years. A 3-year severe narrowing of proximal right and left ACAs and left MCA. (b) At seven years of age, occlusion of left MCA and both ACAs and extensive bilateral lenticulostriate perforator collaterals and left cerebellar collaterals (arrows) suggestive of a Moya network. (c) At seven years of age, FLAIR axial view. Sequelae of the left internal borderzone infarct.

called kinkings that are more prevalent than in the general population and evolve over time as a function of the degree of anemia and eICA-TAMVs [44]. This favors a remodeling mechanism as a consequence of high blood flow associated with severe chronic anemia. Extracranial ICA arteriopathy can affect the entire course of the ICAs with a more severe evolution of proximal web-like lesions (**Figure 11**) [44].

5.2 Incidence of stenoses during aging

In the Créteil cohort, cerebral MRI/MRA has been systematically performed since 1992, every 2 years since age 5 or earlier in children placed on chronic transfusion for abnormally high cerebral velocities and was available in 375 SCD children. Neck MRA was added in 2011 [19].

5.2.1 Incidence of intracranial stenosis

No SC/Sb + child developed intracranial stenosis during infancy, while intracranial stenosis was detected in 37/332 (11.1%) MRA-assessed SCA children, in which 31 had a history of intracranial abnormal velocities. Among the six children without abnormal intracranial velocities, five had history of conditional velocities and one had no available temporal window.

The presence of intracranial stenosis was highly significantly associated with a history of abnormal high intracranial velocities: OR = 13.7 (95%CI: 5.8–32.3), $p < 0.001$ (**Figure 12**).

5.2.2 Incidence of eICA stenosis

No SC/Sb + child developed eICA stenosis, while it was detected in 32/306 (10.5%) SCA children assessed with neck MRA whose 27 had a history of eICA ≥160 cm/s and 30 had eICA kinking. The presence of eICA stenosis was highly significantly and independently associated with a history of eICA TAMV ≥160 cm/s: OR = 15.2 (95%CI: 3.2–71.4), $p < 0.001$ and with the presence of eICA kinking: OR = 15.2 (95%CI: 3.2–71.4), $p = 0.001$. eICA kinking was also significantly associated with the number of SEN-beta-haplotypes: OR = 1.5 (95%CI: 1.04–2.08), $p = 0.028$ (**Figure 13**).

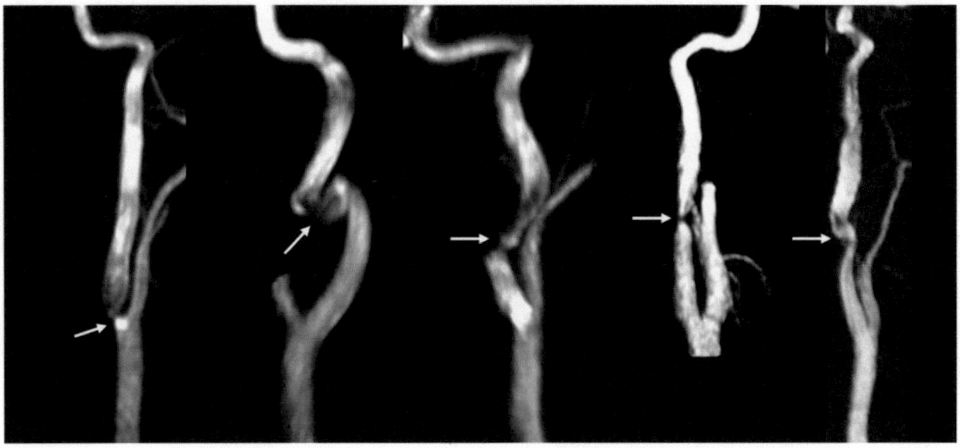

Figure 11.
3D TOF MRA of the cervical ICA after segmentation. Cervical ICA stenosis in five different patients.

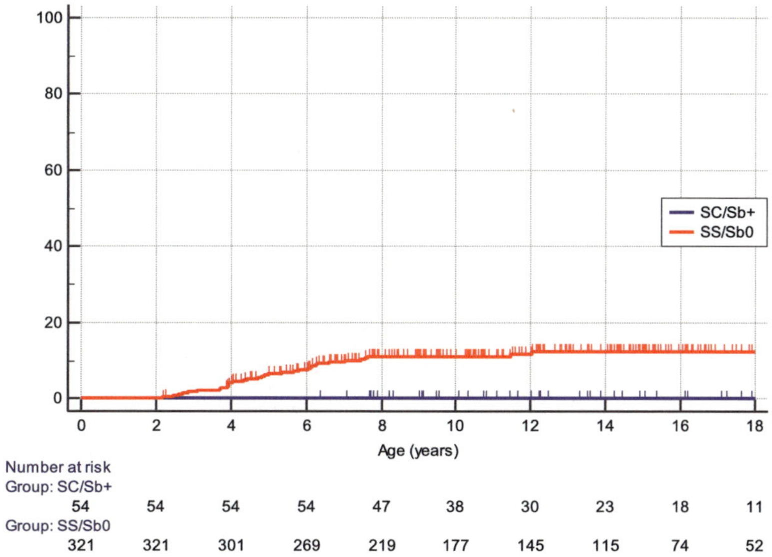

Figure 12.
Cumulative incidence of intracranial stenosis in Créteil SCD cohort: at 10 years of age: 11.1% (95%CI: 7.5–14.7%) in SCA versus 0% in SC/Sb + children (p = 0.001).

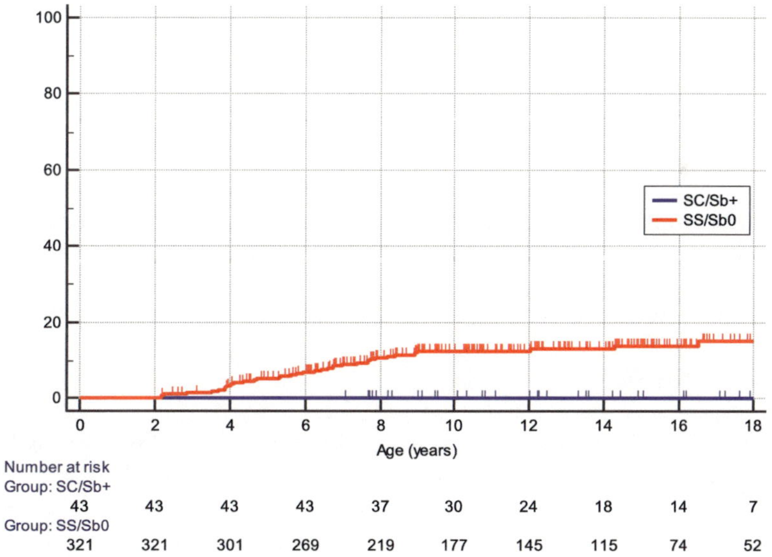

Figure 13.
Cumulative incidence of eICA stenosis in the Créteil SCD cohort: at 10 years of age: 12.3% (95%CI: 8.3–16.3%) in SCA versus 0% in SC/Sb + children (p = 0.015).

5.3 Management of cerebral arterial stenoses

In France, the recommendation for intracranial stenoses is to initiate and maintain chronic transfusion unless there is a possibility of transplantation. In the DREPAGREFFE trial, comparing chronic transfusion to transplantation, among the 67 patients with a history of cerebral TAMV ≥200 cm/s, 60 were stroke-free and 28 of them had stenosis at enrollment: 14 of them were transplanted, while the other 14 children were maintained on chronic transfusion. The outcome of stenosis score was significantly better in the transplanted group than in the transfused group [45].

By contrast, there is no recommendation concerning eICA arteriopathy and the impact of hydroxyurea treatment is unknown. In Debré center, it has been recently shown [44] that eICA stenosis score was more reduced on chronic transfusion than on hydroxyurea or on simple observation.

6. Silent cerebral ischemia (SCI)

6.1 MRI detection of silent cerebral ischemia

Silent cerebral ischemia (SCI) refers to ischemic damage identified on imaging that does not have a clinical correlate. SCI is detected in MRI that is recommended to do systematically from the age of 5 years in SS/Sb0 children when it does not require sedation. It is defined as a hyperintensity focus of at least 3 mm in diameter, visible in two planes on FLAIR MRI [46]. SCI occurs in infants as young as 1 year of age and continue throughout childhood [47].

SCIs reflect the severity of the disease, as they are associated with cognitive impairment, reduced academic achievement [48, 49], and a 14-fold increased risk of overt ischemic stroke [50]. Lesions are mostly confined to the white matter within the frontal and parietal border zone areas. The predilection for these areas is explained by the lower blood supply from end arterioles between the deep and the superficial territory of the MCA and between vascular territories.

6.2 Incidence of SCI

Despite early TCD screening and systematic assessment by cerebral MRI/MRA since age 5, the cumulative incidence of SCIs in the SCA Créteil newborn cohort was 37% by age 14 and did not reach a plateau [17]. This finding was confirmed in an adult series showing a prevalence of 53.3% by age 30 [51]. Contrary to large vessel arteriopathy, only observed in SCA children, SCIs were also observed in SC/Sb + children.

6.3 Risk factors for SCI

Risk factors for SCI are low baseline hemoglobin [17, 52, 53], intracranial and extracranial stenoses [17, 53, 54], relative hypertension, male sex [52], and acute and chronic anemia [53]. As a matter of fact, SCIs are more frequent in the presence of extra and intracranial stenoses [53, 55], but are also seen in the absence of large vessel arteriopathy, suggesting a contribution to tissue-level hypoperfusion and hypoxia, such as during episodes of acute anemia due to splenic sequestration or erythroblastopenia or during episodes of hypoxia during thoracic syndromes.

6.4 Management of SCI

The SIT trial compared in SCA children with SCI the 3-year outcome on chronic transfusion versus simple observation. The recurrence rate was significantly lower on chronic transfusion (p = 0.04) than on simple observation, but the difference between both groups was not enough sufficient to convince practitioners to initiate long-term chronic transfusion with the risks of alloimmunization, blood availability, and iron overload risk. No randomized trial comparing hydroxyurea to simple observation or to chronic transfusion is available. However, SCI being significantly associated with lower cognitive performances and anemia justify to introduce hydroxyurea if not already given. However, several studies have reported SCI occurrence despite ongoing hydroxyurea treatment [56, 57]. Moreover, SCI presence being a marker of SCA-related severity encourages to consider chronic transfusion and to search for an available donor for transplantation [58].

7. Conclusion

Early assessment of children with SCA by transcranial and cervical Doppler ultrasound should be recommended not only to prevent overt but also SCI associated with poor cognitive performance. In addition, brain MRI and neck MRA are recommended to look for ischemic lesions and arterial stenosis and to choose the most appropriate treatment.

Hydroxyurea, by improving anemia and hemolysis, reduces the risk of abnormally high velocity and stroke, but chronic transfusion is still recommended for children identified as being at risk of stroke due to abnormally high brain velocities. A switch from chronic transfusion to hydroxyurea is recommended in children with normalized velocities and no arterial stenosis. However, in the presence of arterial stenosis, chronic transfusion and especially stem cell transplantation are more effective and should be recommended. These recommendations need to be reconsidered in low-income countries, where cost, availability, and safety of blood products are a major limit.

Author details

Françoise Bernaudin* and Suzanne Verlhac
Reference Centre for Sickle Cell Disease, CHIC Hospital, Créteil and Robert Debré Hospital, APHP, Paris, France

*Address all correspondence to: francoise.bernaudin@chicreteil.fr

References

[1] Connes P, Verlhac S, Bernaudin F. Advances in understanding the pathogenesis of cerebrovascular vasculopathy in sickle cell anaemia. British Journal of Haematology. 2013;**161**:484-498

[2] Rothman SM, Fulling KH, Nelson JS. Sickle cell anemia and central nervous system infarction: A neuropathological study. Annals of Neurology. 1986;**20**:684-690

[3] Ohene-Frempong K, Weiner SJ, Sleeper LA, Miller ST, EmburyS,MoohrJW,etal.Cerebrovascular accidents in sickle cell disease: Rates and risk factors. Blood. 1998;**91**:288-294

[4] Gueguen A, Mahevas M, Nzouakou R, Hosseini H, Habibi A, Bachir D, et al. Sickle-cell disease stroke throughout life: A retrospective study in an adult referral center. American Journal of Hematology. 2014;**89**(3):267-272. DOI: 10.1002/ajh.23625

[5] Russell MO, Goldberg HI, Hodson A, Kim HC, Halus J, Reivich M, et al. Effect of transfusion therapy on arteriographic abnormalities and on recurrence of stroke in sickle cell disease. Blood. 1984;**63**:162-169

[6] Hulbert ML, McKinstry RC, Lacey JL, Moran CJ, Panepinto JA, Thompson AA, et al. Silent cerebral infarcts occur despite regular blood transfusion therapy after first strokes in children with sickle cell disease. Blood. 2011;**117**:772-779

[7] Wang WC, Kovnar EH, Tonkin IL, Mulhern RK, Langston JW, Day SW, et al. High risk of recurrent stroke after discontinuance of five to twelve years of transfusion therapy in patients with sickle cell disease. The Journal of Pediatrics. 1991;**118**:377-382

[8] Ware RE, Zimmerman SA, Schultz WH. Hydroxyurea as an alternative to blood transfusions for the prevention of recurrent stroke in children with sickle cell disease. Blood. 1999;**94**:3022-3026

[9] Ware RE, Helms RW, SWiTCH Investigators. Stroke with transfusions changing to hydroxyurea (SWiTCH). Blood. 2012;**119**:3925-3932

[10] Bernaudin F, Verlhac S, Arnaud C, Kamdem A, Hau I, Leveillé E, et al. Long-term treatment follow-up of children with sickle cell disease monitored with abnormal transcranial Doppler velocities. Blood. 2016;**127**:1814-1822

[11] Walters MC, Storb R, Patience M, Leisenring W, Taylor T, Sanders JE, et al. Impact of bone marrow transplantation for symptomatic sickle cell disease: An interim report. Multicenter investigation of bone marrow transplantation for sickle cell disease. Blood. 2000;**95**:1918-1924

[12] Kossorotoff M, Brousse V, Grevent D, et al. Cerebral haemorrhagic risk in children with sickle-cell disease. Developmental Medicine and Child Neurology. 2015;**57**:187-193

[13] Gendreau S, Scholer M, Cecchini J, Habibi A, Razazi K, De Prost N, et al. Cerebral fat embolism in sickle cell disease. American Journal of Hematology. 2020;**95**(2):E41-E45. DOI: 10.1002/ajh.25686

[14] Adams RJ, McKie V, Nichols F, Carl E, Zhang DL, McKie K, et al. The use of transcranial ultrasonography to predict stroke in sickle cell disease.

The New England Journal of Medicine. 1992;**326**:605-610

[15] Adams RJ, McKie VC, Carl EM, Nichols FT, Perry R, Brock K, et al. Long-term stroke risk in children with sickle cell disease screened with transcranial Doppler. Annals of Neurology. 1997;**42**:699-704

[16] Adams RJ, McKie VC, Hsu L, Files B, Vichinsky E, Pegelow C, et al. Prevention of a first stroke by transfusions in children with sickle cell anemia and abnormal results on transcranial Doppler ultrasonography. The New England Journal of Medicine. 1998;**339**:5-11

[17] Bernaudin F, Verlhac S, Arnaud C, Kamdem A, Chevret S, Hau I, et al. Impact of early transcranial Doppler screening and intensive therapy on cerebral vasculopathy outcome in a newborn sickle cell anemia cohort. Blood. 2011;**117**:1130-1140

[18] Verlhac S, Balandra S, Cussenot I, Kasbi F, Vasile M, Kheniche A, et al. Extracranial carotid arteriopathy in stroke-free children with sickle cell anemia: Detection by submandibular Doppler sonography. Pediatric Radiology. 2014;**44**:587-596

[19] Bernaudin F, Verlhac S, Arnaud C, et al. Cumulative incidences and risk factors for intra and extracranial cerebral arteriopathy in sickle cell disease children. Blood. 2020;**136**(S1):56-57

[20] Bernaudin F, Verlhac S, Chevret S, Torres M, Coic L, Arnaud C, et al. G6PD deficiency, absence of alpha-thalassemia, and hemolytic rate at baseline are significant independent risk factors for abnormally high cerebral velocities in patients with sickle cell anemia. Blood. 2008;**112**:4314-4317

[21] Charache S, Dover GJ, Moore RD, et al. Hydroxyurea: Effects on hemoglobin F production in patients with sickle cell anemia. Blood. 1992;**79**(10):2555-2565

[22] Wang WC, Ware RE, Miller ST, et al. BABY HUG investigators. Hydroxycarbamide in very young children with sickle-cell anaemia: A multicentre, randomised, controlled trial (BABY HUG). Lancet. 2011;**377**(9778):1663-1672

[23] Opoka RO, Ndugwa CM, Latham TS, et al. Novel use of hydroxyurea in an african region with malaria (NOHARM): A trial for children with sickle cell anemia. Blood. 2017;**130**(24):2585-2593

[24] Tshilolo L, Tomlinson G, Williams TN, et al. REACH Investigators. Hydroxyurea for children with sickle cell Anemia in sub-Saharan Africa. The New England Journal of Medicine. 2019;**380**(2):121-131

[25] Zimmerman SA, Schultz WH, Burgett S, Mortier NA, Ware RE. Hydroxyurea therapy lowers transcranial Doppler flow velocities in children with sickle cell anemia. Blood. 2007;**110**(3):1043-1047

[26] Lagunju I, Brown BJ, Sodeinde O. Hydroxyurea lowers transcranial Doppler flow velocities in children with sickle cell anaemia in a Nigerian cohort. Pediatric Blood & Cancer. 2015;**62**(9):1587-1591

[27] Adegoke SA, Macedo-Campos RS, Braga JAP, Figueiredo MS, Silva GS. Changes in transcranial Doppler flow velocities in children with sickle cell disease: The impact of hydroxyurea therapy. Journal of Stroke and Cerebrovascular Diseases. 2018;**27**(2):425-431

[28] Lagunju I, Brown BJ, Oyinlade AO, et al. Annual stroke incidence in Nigerian

children with sickle cell disease and elevated TCD velocities treated with hydroxyurea. Pediatric Blood & Cancer. 2019;**66**(3):e27252

[29] Galadanci NA, Umar Abdullahi S, Vance LD, et al. Feasibility trial for primary stroke prevention in children with sickle cell anemia in Nigeria (SPIN trial). American Journal of Hematology. 2017;**92**:780-788

[30] Galadanci NA, Abdullahi SU, Shehi Ali Abubakar SA, et al. Moderate fixed-dose hydroxyurea for primary prevention of strokes in Nigerian children with sickle cell disease: Final results of the SPIN trial. American Journal of Hematology. 2020;**95**(9):E247-E250

[31] Thornburg CD, Files BA, Luo Z, et al. Impact of hydroxyurea on clinical events in the BABY HUG trial. Blood. 2012;**120**(22):4304-4310 quiz 4448

[32] Hankins JS, McCarville MB, Rankine-Mullings A, et al. Prevention of conversion to abnormal transcranial Doppler with hydroxyurea in sickle cell anemia: A phase III international randomized clinical trial. American Journal of Hematology. 2015;**90**(12):1099-1105

[33] Opoka RO, Hume HA, Latham TS, et al. Hydroxyurea to lower transcranial Doppler velocities and prevent primary stroke: The Uganda NOHARM sickle cell anemia cohort. Haematologica. 2020;**105**(6):e272-e275

[34] Yawn BP, Buchanan GR, Afenyi-Annan AN, et al. Management of sickle cell disease: Summary of the 2014 evidence-based report by expert panel members. Journal of the American Medical Association. 2014;**312**(10):1033-1048

[35] Vichinsky E, Hoppe CC, Ataga KI, et al. HOPE trial Investigators. A phase 3 randomized trial of Voxelotor in sickle cell disease. The New England Journal of Medicine. 2019;**381**(6):509-519

[36] Adams RJ. Brambilla D of the STOP 2 investigative team. Discontinuing prophylactic transfusions used to prevent stroke in sickle cell disease. The New England Journal of Medicine. 2005;**353**:2769-2778

[37] Bernaudin F, Verlhac S, Coïc L, Lesprit E, Brugières P, Reinert P. Long term follow-up of pediatric sickle cell disease patients with abnormal high velocities on transcranial Doppler. Pediatric Radiology. 2005;**35**(3):242-248

[38] Ware RE, Davis BR, Schultz WH, Brown RC, Aygun B, Sarnaik S, et al. Hydroxycarbamide versus chronic transfusion for maintenance of transcranial doppler flow velocities in children with sickle cell anaemia-TCD with transfusions changing to hydroxyurea (TWiTCH): A multicentre, open-label, phase 3, non-inferiority trial. Lancet. 2016;**387**:661-670

[39] Bernaudin F, Verlhac S, Peffault de Latour R, Dalle JH, Brousse V, Petras E, et al. Association of Matched Sibling Donor Hematopoietic Stem Cell Transplantation with Transcranial Doppler Velocities in children with sickle cell Anemia. JAMA. 2019;**321**:266-276

[40] Brewin J, Kaya B, Chakravorty S. How I manage sickle cell patients with high transcranial doppler results. British Journal of Haematology. 2017;**179**(3):377-388

[41] DeBaun MR, Jordan LC, King AA, et al. American Society of Hematology 2020 guidelines for sickle cell disease: Prevention, diagnosis, and

treatment of cerebrovascular disease in children and adults. Blood Advances. 2020;**4**(8):1554-1588

[42] Loggetto SR, Veríssimo MPA, Darrigo-Junior LG, Simões RDS, Bernardo WM, Braga JAP. Guidelines on sickle cell disease: Primary stroke prevention in children and adolescents. Hematology Transfusion and Cell Therapy. 2022;**44**(1):85-94

[43] Kandeel AY, Zimmerman RA, Ohene-Frempong K. Comparison of magnetic resonance angiography and conventional angiography in sickle cell disease: Clinical significance and reliability. Neuroradiology. 1996;**38**(5):409-416

[44] Verlhac S, Ithier G, Bernaudin F, Oloukoi C, Cussenot I, Balandra S, et al. Evolution of extracranial internal carotid artery disease in children with sickle cell anemia. Stroke. 2022. DOI: 10.1161. Online ahead of print

[45] Verlhac S, Gabor F, Paillard C, et al. Improved stenosis outcome in stroke-free sickle cell anemia children after transplantation compared to chronic transfusion. British Journal of Haematology. 2021;**193**(1):188-193

[46] DeBaun MR, Gordon M, McKinstry RC, Noetzel MJ, White DA, Sarnaik SA, et al. Controlled trial of transfusions for silent cerebral infarcts in sickle cell anemia. The New England Journal of Medicine. 2014;**371**:699-710

[47] Wang WC, Pavlakis SG, Helton KJ, McKinstry RC, Casella JF, Adams RJ, et al. MRI abnormalities of the brain in one-year-old children with sickle cell anemia. Pediatric Blood & Cancer. 2008;**51**(5):643-646

[48] DeBaun MR, Schatz J, Siegel MJ, Koby M, Craft S, Resar L, et al. Cognitive screening examinations for silent cerebral infarcts in sickle cell disease. Neurology. 1998;**50**:1678-1682

[49] Bernaudin F, Verlhac S, Fréard F, Roudot-Thoraval F, Benkerrou M, Thuret I, et al. Multicenter prospective study of children with sickle cell disease: Radiographic and psychometric correlation. Journal of Child Neurology. 2000;**15**:333-343

[50] Miller ST, Macklin EA, Pegelow CH, Kinney TR, Sleeper LA, Bello JA, et al. Silent infarction as a risk factor for overt stroke inchildren with sickle cell anemia: A report from the cooperative study of sickle cell disease. The Journal of Pediatrics. 2001;**139**:385-390

[51] Kassim AA, Pruthi S, Day M, Rodeghier M, Gindville MC, Brodsky MA, et al. Silent cerebral infarcts and cerebral aneurysms are prevalent in adults with sickle cell anemia. Blood. 2016;**127**:2038-2040

[52] DeBaun MR, Sarnaik SA, Rodeghier MJ, Minniti CP, Howard TH, Iyer RV, et al. Associated risk factors for silent cerebral infarcts in sickle cell anemia: Low baseline hemoglobin, sex, and relative high systolic blood pressure. Blood. 2012;**119**:3684-3690

[53] Bernaudin F, Verlhac S, Arnaud C, Kamdem A, Vasile M, Kasbi F, et al. Chronic and acute anemia and extracranial internal carotid stenosis are risk factors for silent cerebral infarcts in sickle cell anemia. Blood. 2015;**125**:1653-1661

[54] Kwiatkowski JL, Zimmerman RA, Pollock AN, Seto W, Smith-Whitley K, Shults J, et al. Silent infarcts in young children with sickle cell disease. British Journal of Haematology. 2009;**146**:300-305

[55] Thangarajh M, Yang G, Fuchs D, et al. Magnetic resonance angiography-defined intracranial vasculopathy is associated with silent cerebral infarcts and glucose-6-phosphate dehydrogenase mutation in children with sickle cell anaemia. British Journal of Haematology. 2012;**159**(3):352-359

[56] Nottage KA, Ware RE, Aygun B, Smeltzer M, Kang G, Moen J, et al. Hydroxycarbamide treatment and brain MRI/MRA findings in children with sickle cell anaemia. British Journal of Haematology. 2016;**175**:331-338

[57] Rushton T, Aban I, Young D, Howard T, Hilliard L, Lebensburger J. Hydroxycarbamide for patients with silent cerebral infarcts: Outcomes and patient preference. British Journal of Haematology. 2018;**181**:145-148

[58] Bernaudin F. What is the place of hematopoietic stem cell transplantation in the management of cerebral vasculopathy in children with sickle cell anemia? Hematology/Oncology and Stem Cell Therapy. 2020;**13**(3):121-130

Chapter 4

Kidney Injuries in Sickle Cell Disease

Samit Ghosh

Abstract

Sickle cell disease (SCD), characterized by the presence of unstable sickle hemoglobin in the homozygous state (HbSS), results in progressive organ damage and early mortality with the median age of death in the 40s. The kidney is one of the most severely affected organs in SCD. Kidney diseases gradually develop in individuals with SCD. Microalbuminuria is evident in childhood, progressing to apparent proteinuria, deteriorating glomerular filtration rate (GFR) in early adulthood. While CKD becomes prevalent in adults. Moreover, among SCD patients, exacerbation of anemia is an independent risk factor for acute kidney injury (AKI) which is a predisposing factor for CKD and End Stage Renal Diseases (ESRD), altogether contributing to 16–18% mortality among this patients' population. The pathogenesis of renal diseases in SCD is not completely understood. While epidemiological studies have shown a strong association between rate of hemolysis, severity of anemia and CKD, intrinsic inflammatory, oxidative and hypercoagulative stress that contribute to the characteristic endothelial dysfunction also promotes development of renal diseases in SCD. This chapter will elaborately discuss current research on the pathogenesis of AKI, AKI-to-CKD transition and future research perspectives for development of novel therapeutic strategies.

Keywords: sickle cell disease, hemolysis, endothelium, AKI, CKD

1. Introduction

Kidney diseases are a major clinical concern in sickle cell disorders (SCD). Acute kidney injury (AKI) as well as chronic kidney disease (CKD) is associated with higher risk of inpatient mortality, prolonged hospital stay and expensive hospitalizations [1, 2]. While an estimated 100,000 people are affected by SCD in the United States (US) [3–5], about 20–25 million people are living with SCD worldwide and the number is expected to increase by about 30% globally by 2050 [6]. In the US, the majority of healthcare for SCD is attributed to in-patient hospitalization for acute complications with an estimated annual cost of $953,640 per patient per year [7]. Progressive kidney disease leads to significant morbidity and mortality in both pediatric and adult patients with SCD. Sickle cell nephropathy (SCN) comprehends a spectrum of renal abnormalities that begins in childhood and may progress to advanced renal disorders in adulthood. In contrast to mild renal manifestations of sickle cell nephropathy includes decreased urinary concentrating ability, impaired renal acidification and potassium secretion, hematuria and proteinuria, progressive kidney disease leads to significant morbidity and mortality in both pediatric and adult patients with SCD. Acute Kidney Injury (AKI) causes sudden drop in kidney function and promotes chronic kidney disease (CKD) and end stage renal disease (ESRD) [8–10]. In SCD, incidences of AKI are common among hospitalized SCD patients [11–13] and it is associated with increased mortality in those admitted to intensive care unit [14]. It is also an independent risk factor for increase morbidity, longer hospitalizations, and increased costs [15] as well as with risk for CKD progression in SCD [16]. Approximately 30% of SCD individuals develop CKD by adulthood and a large proportion of this sub-population develops ESRD [17]. The annual rate of incidence of AKI and reported CKD is 2–3-fold higher among SCD patients compared to non-sickle individuals [2]. Although newborn screening along with early intervention decreased early childhood mortality in SCD, accumulation of kidney diseases and age dependent renal deterioration of renal health poses increased risk of mortality in this population.

2. SCD pathophysiology and susceptibility to acute kidney injury

The genetic basis of SCD includes a single point mutation in the beta-globin chain of hemoglobin resulting in a morphologically and functionally different red blood cells (RBC). The modified hemoglobin (HbS) polymerizes under hypoxic condition causing RBC sickling [18, 19]. This characteristic feature of SCD leads to two major pathophysiological consequences, namely, vasoocclusion and hemolysis [20]. Moreover renal medullary hypoxia, acidosis, hyperosmolarity and reduced blood flow contribute to elevated endothelial adhesion and recurrent ischemia–reperfusion (IR) injury [13]. Earlier studies implicated several aspects of SCD including volume depletion, rhabdomyolysis, infections and the use of non-steroidal analgesics (NSAIDs) as predisposing factors for AKI [13, 21–25]. A cascade of these events individually or in combination possibly generates a constellation of sterile inflammation and oxidative stress, which overwhelm the normal physiology and trigger several chronic and acute multiorgan damage including kidney injury in SCD. Recurrent episodes of IR injury trigger vasoocclusive pain crisis (VOC), one of the major causes for intensive care unit (ICU) admission for patients with SCD. This medically vulnerable population is at higher risk of developing AKI due to co-morbid conditions of kidney and other organs including heart and lung. Patients with SCD frequently develop cardiopulmonary events like pulmonary hypertension (PH) and acute chest syndrome (ACS) which often lead to premature death [26]. AKI is emerging as a major clinical concern among SCD patients hospitalized for VOC and acute chest syndrome (ACS). It has been reported in ~14% of adults [12] and 8% children [27] with ACS, and in 17% of children with VOC [28]. Additionally, while hyperfiltration and microalbuminuria are common in SCD [13], chronic kidney disease (CKD) occurs in up to 60% of these patients [17]. Recent epidemiological evidences increasingly indicate that CKD and AKI are linked and probably promote one another [29, 30]. Underlying CKD is now recognized as a clear risk factor for AKI, as both decreased glomerular filtration rate (GFR) and increased proteinuria.

2.1 Hemolysis and acute kidney injury in SCD

Acute exacerbation of anemia that potentially generate excess extracellular heme is an independent risk factor for AKI in SCD [27, 28, 31]. Earlier studies implicated several aspects of SCD including volume depletion, rhabdomyolysis, infections and the use of non-steroidal analgesics (NSAIDs) as predisposing factors for AKI [13, 21–25]. Recent clinical studies have concluded that incidences of AKI are associated with rapid decline in hemoglobin (Hb). The link between acute hemolysis and AKI is corroborated with significantly low level of total Hb at the time of hospitalization among SCD patients who develop AKI compared to those who do not [16], and higher risk of developing acute renal insufficiency among ACS patients with rapidly progressive decline in total Hb [32]. Intravascular hemolysis is a cardinal pathophysiological event in SCD that raises cell free plasma Hb and arginase-1 levels to collectively reduce nitric oxide (NO) bioavailability and enhance reactive oxygen species (ROS) formation [33, 34]. Cell-free hemoglobin is primarily scavenged by plasma protein haptoglobin (Hp). The resulting duo (Hb-Hp complex) is internalized by macrophage receptor CD163 for subsequent globin and heme metabolism. Haptoglobin is depleted in SCD resulting high amount of plasma hemoglobin that can easily get exposed to the underlying oxidative environment. Heme is subsequently released following oxidation of Hb to methemoglobin (metHb) with ferric heme. Extracellular circulating heme is rapidly transferred to hemopexin (Hx), the plasma protein with the highest binding affinity for heme. It is well known that heme-hemopexin (heme-Hx) complex is transported to the liver for degradation by heme oxygenase-1 (HO-1) [35, 36]. In SCD, plasma Hx is also intrinsically exhausted due to chronic hemolysis [37, 38]. Lack of haptoglobin and hemopexin along with chronic and acute hemolysis elevate extracellular hemoglobin and heme in plasma of SCD patients [33]. Furthermore, the HbS is a relatively unstable molecule that can easily undergo autooxidation contributing to increase circulating free heme in SCD [39]. Both cell-free circulating hemoglobin and heme are toxic, unless sufficiently metabolized, to the cells and may cause significant damage to organs including kidney.

2.2 Pathogenesis of acute kidney injury in SCD

The primary etiology of AKI involves four major structures of kidney including tubules, glomeruli, interstitium and intrarenal blood vessels. While acute tubular injury is the major pathological manifestation of AKI, rapid decline in renal function identified by reduced glomerular filtration rate (GFR) clinically define AKI [40]. The dimeric form of circulating cell free Hb can filter through glomerular sieve and enters in proximal tubular segment. The endocytosis of Hb molecules is possible through the megalin and cubilin receptors on tubular epithelial cells. The internalized hemoglobin breaks down in to heme that induces caspase-3 mediated apoptosis of the tubular cells leading to AKI development. This idea was supported by the presence of hemoglobin and myoglobin in plasma and urinary space in multiple in vivo models of AKI induced by glycerol, ischemia, sepsis and cisplatin [41–43].

In vivo, excess circulating heme, a byproduct of acute hemolysis, triggers VOC and ACS, the two major SCD complications associated with hospitalization and AKI development in SCD [44, 45]. Our recent study demonstrated that modest elevation of extracellular heme in circulation promotes clinically relevant AKI in an established humanized murine model of SCD containing human HbS. In this study, the researchers have established that a secondary heme scavenger, alpha-1-microglobin (A1M) is elevated in mice and human with SCD as an adaptive response to decreased hemopexin, the primary heme scavenger responsible for clearance of circulating free heme [46]. Several other studies have shown that heme bound to A1M is transported to renal tubular epithelial cells [47]. Excess deposition of heme causes proximal tubular

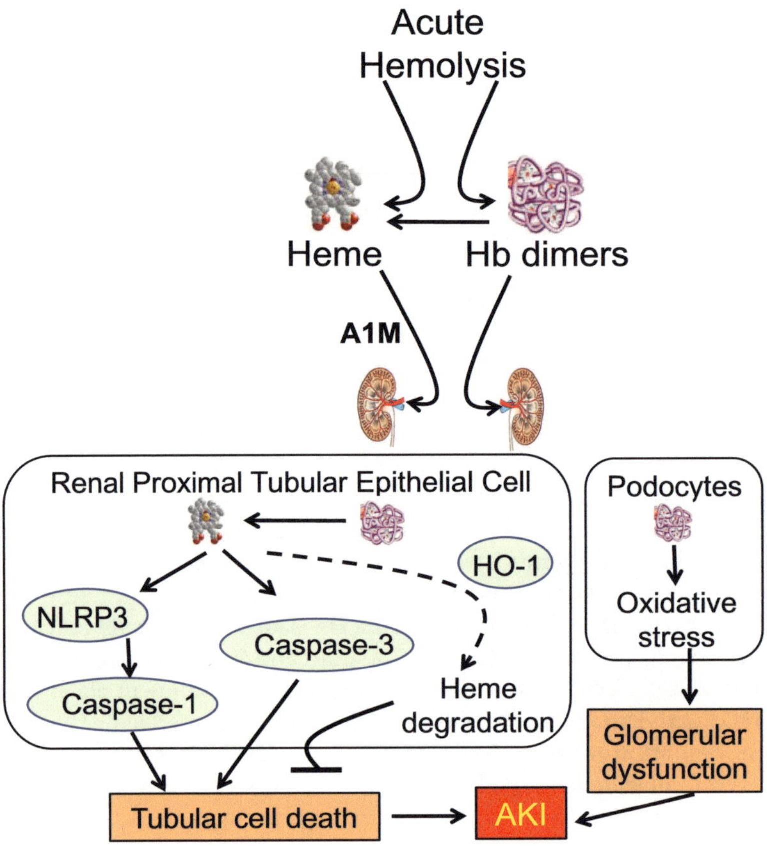

Figure 1.
Pathogenesis of AKI in SCD. Hemolysis cause release of cell free Hb and heme in circulation. Free dimeric Hb or free heme bound to A1M passes through glomerular filtration and internalized into renal proximal tubular epithelial cells. Excess heme can overwhelm the HO-1 degradation capacity and induce multiple cell death pathways. On the other hand, Hb may cause podocyte injury leading to glomerular dysfunction. Tubular cell death and/or glomerular damage develops AKI.

epithelial cell death and promotes AKI (**Figure 1**). This study identifies that relative concentration of A1M and Hx may serve as prognostic factor of future AKI events in SCD during acute hemolytic events [46, 48].

3. Chronic kidney disease (CKD) in sickle cell disorders

Kidney diseases gradually develop in individuals with SCD. Microalbuminuria is evident in childhood, progressing to apparent proteinuria, deteriorating glomerular filtration rate (GFR) in early adulthood, while CKD becomes prevalent in adults [49]. Development of CKD in SCD is complex, but several studies have invariably demonstrated its association with low hemoglobin level and hemolysis [50–53]. Higher frequency of severe anemia (Hb: 7–9 g/dl) among SCD patients with ESRD (71%) compared to non-SCD patients with ESRD (25%) has also been reported [54]. Moreover, among SCD patients, exacerbation of anemia is an independent risk factor for acute kidney injury (AKI) which is a predisposing factor for CKD and ESRD [27, 28, 31]. Progression of kidney damage is defined as CKD when eGFR is reduced to

<60 mL/min/1.73 m^2. The reduced GFR is often associated with hematuria, albuminuria and nephrotic syndromes. Intravascular hemolysis is a cardinal pathophysiological event in SCD that raises cell free plasma hemoglobin and arginase 1 to collectively reduce nitric oxide (NO) bioavailability and enhance reactive oxygen species (ROS) formation [33, 34]. Worsening anemia and elevated persistent oxidative stress lead to decline in GFR in association with reduced erythropoietin synthesis. Individuals with SCD develop CKD at a median age of 23.1 years, while 16–27% of pediatric patients have CKD [17].

3.1 Glomerular hyperfiltration, hyper perfusion and progressive kidney damage

Increased renal blood flow and higher GFR are characteristics of kidney function among SCD patients at their younger age. The hyperfiltration subsides to normal GFR that eventually lowers to subnormal level with the progression of age and the development of CKD [13, 55]. Sustained glomerular hyperfiltration causes damage to different parts of the glomerulus including the endothelium and the epithelial layer of the Bowman's capsule. These events predispose the development of focal segmental glomerular sclerosis (FSGS), which is a common feature in SCD. Hyperfiltration occurs due to glomerular hyper perfusion that increases the renal blood flow. Hyper perfusion stems from underlying anemia and decreased vascular resistance, while the reduced blood flow is evident within hypoxic renal medulla due to vasoocclusion of sickle red blood cells. This phenomenon commonly known as "perfusion paradox" generates increased oxidative stress, mesangial proliferation, endothelial barrier disruption, and thickening of the glomerular basement membrane [56].

3.2 Proteinuria and chronic kidney disease in SCD

Hyperfiltration among children with SCD is associated with proteinuria in the form of microalbuminuria (urine albumin 30–300 mg/g creatinine). This condition increases with age and about 68% of these patients experienced macroalbuminuria (urine albumin >300 mg/g creatinine) as they grow older [57, 58]. While about 4% of SCD patients exhibit macroalbuminuria at the nephrotic range (urine albumin >500 mg/g creatinine), a substantial number of patients suffer from irreversible kidney complications. Several studies have indicated association of albuminuria with hemolysis, incidences of vasoocclusive crisis and acute chest syndrome, and pulmonary hypertension. These events also impact blood pressure which in turn can regulate hyperfiltration [13, 17, 21, 53].

3.3 Genetic variants associated with chronic kidney disease in SCD

Apart from the underlying hemoglobin gene mutation, progression and severity of CKD development are associated with polymorphisms of multiples genes among SCD patients. A major proportion of SCD population has alpha thalassemia. Two polymorphisms in the α-chain of the globin chain including i) a 3.7 Kb deletion and ii) a 4.2 Kb deletion are associated with reduced albuminuria, higher eGFR and hence lower risk of CKD progression [59, 60].

The variants of apolipoprotein L1 gene (*APOL1)* gene associated with risk of CKD development have been studied widely. The G1 (S342G and I384M) as well as G2 (N388 and Y389 deletion) variants found in 11–13% of African Americans account for about 70% CKD risk in this population. Homozygous or compound heterozygous inheritance of G1/G2 variants within SCD population increase the macroalbuminuria, progression of CKD and development of ESRD [61–63].

Besides the increased risk of AKI with longer GT tandem repeats of HMOX-1 gene promoter, the allele frequency of a variant of *HMOX-1* (rs743811) was found to be associated with worsening CKD [61, 64]. Several other genetic variants including (i) Duffy antigen (Fy rs2814778) of the RBC, (ii) myosin heavy chain 9 (*MYH9*-rs5750248, rs1192763), (iii) *TGF-β/BMP* (BMPR1B) have also been implicated with CKD risk among various cohorts of SCD patients [65–67].

3.4 Renal endothelium and pathogenesis of chronic kidney disease in SCD

In SCD, intrinsic hemolytic, inflammatory, oxidative and hypercoagulative stress contribute to the characteristic endothelial dysfunction that alters the systemic vascular biology [68]. Endothelial interaction with multiple blood components, including sickled red blood cells, leukocytes and platelets, injure the endothelium and obstruct the vasculature impacting internal organs [69]. Renal pathology in sickle cell nephropathy includes extensive peritubular microvascular congestions and chronic thrombotic microangiopathy that can lead to CKD by peritubular microvascular rarefaction, interstitial fibrosis and tubular atrophy [70–72].

Several studies including ours have demonstrated that extracellular heme triggers endothelial barrier disruption in various organs in SCD including the kidneys [44, 73–76]. Endothelial dysfunction may occur in the glomerulus affecting the podocytes that maintain the glomerular endothelial integrity. One study has shown that renal endothelial dysfunction is triggered by an increase in soluble fms-like tyrosine kinase 1 (sFLT-1), a splice variant of vascular endothelial growth factor receptor-1 (VEGFR1) in SCD. The sFLT-1 blocks interaction of VEGF with glomerular endothelium leading to endothelial damage associated with increased albuminuria [77]. Moreover, endothelin-1 (ET-1) generated by endothelial cells under inflammation causes endothelial injury by reducing NO bioavailability. Alongside, ET-1 mediates podocyte injury by binding endothelin A (ETA) receptor. In animal studies, antagonists to ETA receptor showed renal protection [78, 79].

Hemolysis and hemoglobinuria, cardinal features of SCD are associated with proteinuria and progression of CKD in SCD patients [51, 53]. Multiple chronic and acute hemolytic events may induce episodes of vasoocclusion leading to vulnerability of the endothelium susceptible to injury. The peritubular capillaries may split leading hematuria through extravasation of RBCs. These events may prompt development of vasoocclusion of vasa recta and papillary necrosis [80].

Endothelial injury in the renal peritubular microvessels is closely linked to rarefaction and interstitial fibrosis that leads to CKD progression [81–83]. Moreover, free heme reflects the function of danger associated molecular pattern in hemolytic diseases activating vital defense response compartments including toll-like receptor-4 signaling, neutrophil extracellular trap formation and inflammasome activation [84–86]. The inflammatory milieu including activated neutrophils regulate endothelial barrier function through adhesion and secretion dependent mechanisms [87].

4. Current management and therapies

Medications and timely management are critical in protecting the kidney. Chronic RBC transfusion therapy is offered to enhance the osmolality and concentrating ability in children with SCD. Hydroxyurea therapy has been shown to reduce the hyperfiltration in children [88]. Hypotonic fluid is recommended for renal papillary necrosis thiazide or loop diuretics are used to maintain urine flow rate [80]. The angiotensin converting enzyme inhibitors (ACE-inhibitors) can dilate efferent arterioles and help decrease glomerular pressure. ACE-inhibitors are used widely to control albuminuria [89].

5. Future research perspectives

Free heme is considered as an eDAMP (erythroid danger-associated molecular pattern) that induces sterile inflammation in SCD. Heme has been shown to activate toll-like receptor 4 (TLR4) on endothelial cell surface to promote TNFα stimulating innate immune signaling in SCD [45]. Moreover, heme activates NLRP3 inflammasome pathway and releases caspase-1 induced IL-1β from macrophages. The resulting inflammation is associated with hemolysis induced lethality in SCD mice and heme induced cell death in macrophages [85]. Heme-mediated toxicity is particularly relevant to renal tubular epithelial cells as these cells presumably confront the majority of heme that passes through the glomeruli during acute hemolysis. Inflammasomes potentially activate caspase-1 that mediates cell death leading to release of IL-1β and IL-18. These are pro-inflammatory cytokines that are induced and cleaved in the proximal tubule, and subsequently easily detected in the urine of SCD patients and their concentrations were associated with hemolysis [90]. In a cross-sectional study, urine IL-18 levels were markedly elevated in patients with established AKI [91]. An in vitro study using immortalized human proximal tubular epithelial cells (HK-2) suggests that activation of inflammasomes mediates contrast-induced AKI [92]. Whether acute hemolytic events followed by exposure of excess heme on proximal tubular epithelial cell surface induces AKI facilitated by stimulation of inflammasome machinery has not yet been established.

The role of the rate limiting heme catabolizing enzyme, HO-1 may be of significant importance. HO-1 degrades heme into iron (Fe), carbon monoxide (CO) and biliverdin, and thereby protects against adverse effects of heme. Multiple studies featured rapid induction of HO-1 under oxidative stress accounts for its beneficial effect against kidney injury [93–95]. Moreover, longer [GT]n repeats in HO-1 gene (*HMOX1*) promoter, responsible for reduced HO-1 expression, is associated with increased risk of AKI in sickle cell disease patients [16]. The mechanism of cellular regulation of HO-1 induction during AKI events in SCD has yet to be elucidated.

Besides tubular damage, etiology of AKI also includes impaired glomerular structure. Podocytes, the highly differentiated visceral epithelial cells, is a major constituent of glomerular structure and function. One in vitro study has shown that human and murine podocytes exposed to Hb develops increased oxidative stress and undergo apoptosis resulting podocyte dysfunction [96]. In SCD, the cell free HbS may serve as an oxidant to cause podocyte injury that may contributes to AKI, whereas, multiple AKI events may induce focal segmental glomerulosclerosis (FSGS), a characteristic CKD feature in SCD.

The intracellular signaling within the podocyte regulating glomerular endothelial integrity has not been explained.

Despite clinical association, mechanistic studies linking hemolysis to renal peritubular endothelial impairment leading to progressive kidney diseases in SCD have not yet been described. The underlying chronic inflammation in SCD leads to activation

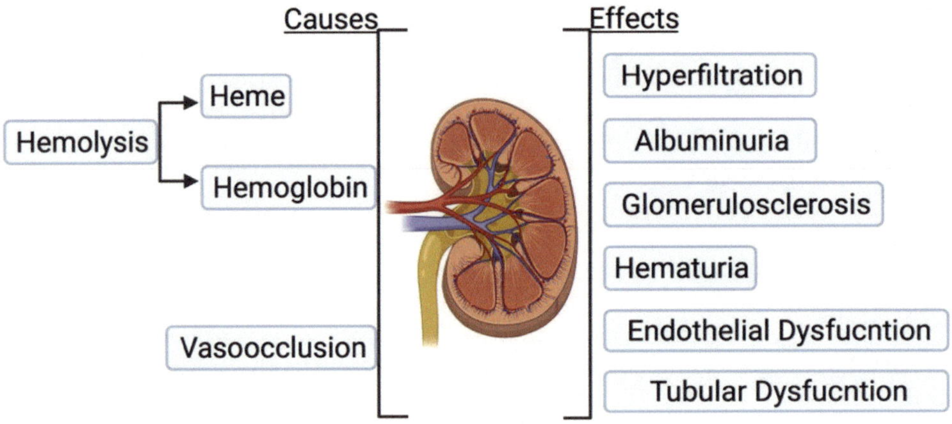

Figure 2.
Overview of sickle cell disease nephropathy. Figure prepared with biorender.com.

of blood cells including neutrophils and platelets. During AKI and CKD, neutrophil and platelet accumulation are evident within renal vasculature. The cellular and molecular mechanism depicting the interactions of activated blood cells and the endothelium leading to progression of CKD is an important area of future research.

Kidney injuries in SCD is multifactorial and may involve multiple unique and overlapping cell biological events in several renal compartments (**Figure 2**). Incidences of AKI are generally considered as independent risk factor for CKD progression not only in general population but also in SCD. Multiple AKI events attributed to acute intravascular hemolytic events in SCD may be responsible for progressive CKD and end stage renal disease among SCD patients. Future studies elucidating mechanisms of AKI to CKD transition along with identification of specific risk factors are warranted for development of potential therapeutics to protect individuals with SCD from broad spectrum of renal complications.

Acknowledgements

Samit Ghosh is supported in part by National Institute of Diabetes and Digestive and Kidney Diseases (NIDDK) [grant R01DK124426]. The author acknowledges research support from Vascular Medicine Institute, the Hemophilia Center of Western Pennsylvania and Vitalant.

Author details

Samit Ghosh
Division of Hematology/Oncology, Department of Medicine, Pittsburgh Heart Lung and Blood Vascular Medicine Institute (VMI), University of Pittsburgh, Pittsburgh, PA, USA

*Address all correspondence to: sag130@pitt.edu

References

[1] Ballas SK. The cost of health care for patients with sickle cell disease. American Journal of Hematology. 2009;**84**(6):320-322

[2] Yeruva SL et al. Renal failure in sickle cell disease: Prevalence, predictors of disease, mortality and effect on length of hospital stay. Hemoglobin. 2016;**40**(5):295-299

[3] Weatherall DJ. Genomics and global health: Time for a reappraisal. Science. 2003;**302**(5645):597-599

[4] Weatherall DJ. Hemoglobinopathies worldwide: Present and future. Current Molecular Medicine. 2008;**8**(7):592-599

[5] Piel FB et al. Global epidemiology of sickle haemoglobin in neonates: A contemporary geostatistical model-based map and population estimates. Lancet. 2013;**381**(9861):142-151

[6] Piel FB et al. Global burden of sickle cell anaemia in children under five, 2010-2050: Modelling based on demographics, excess mortality, and interventions. PLoS Medicine. 2013;**10**(7):e1001484

[7] Kauf TL et al. The cost of health care for children and adults with sickle cell disease. American Journal of Hematology. 2009;**84**(6):323-327

[8] Chawla LS et al. Acute kidney injury and chronic kidney disease as interconnected syndromes. The New England Journal of Medicine. 2014;**371**(1):58-66

[9] Leung KC, Tonelli M, James MT. Chronic kidney disease following acute kidney injury-risk and outcomes. Nature Reviews: Nephrology. 2013;**9**(2):77-85

[10] Venkatachalam MA et al. Acute kidney injury: A springboard for progression in chronic kidney disease. American Journal of Physiology: Renal Physiology. 2010;**298**(5):F1078-F1094

[11] Sklar AH et al. Acute renal failure in sickle cell anemia. The International Journal of Artificial Organs. 1990; **13**(6):347-351

[12] Audard V et al. Acute kidney injury in sickle patients with painful crisis or acute chest syndrome and its relation to pulmonary hypertension. Nephrology, Dialysis, Transplantation. 2010;**25**(8):2524-2529

[13] Nath KA, Hebbel RP. Sickle cell disease: Renal manifestations and mechanisms. Nature Reviews: Nephrology. 2015;**11**(3):161-171

[14] Cecchini J et al. Outcomes of adult patients with sickle cell disease admitted to the ICU: A case series*. Critical Care Medicine. 2014;**42**(7):1629-1639

[15] McCormick M et al. Acute kidney injury in paediatric patients with sickle cell disease is associated with increased morbidity and resource utilization. British Journal of Haematology. 2020;**189**(3):559-565

[16] Saraf SL et al. HMOX1 and acute kidney injury in sickle cell anemia. Blood. 2018;**132**(15):1621-1625

[17] Powars DR et al. Chronic renal failure in sickle cell disease: Risk factors, clinical course, and mortality. Annals of Internal Medicine. 1991;**115**(8):614-620

[18] Bunn HF. Pathogenesis and treatment of sickle cell disease. The New England Journal of Medicine. 1997;**337**(11):762-769

[19] Pauling L and ITANO HA. Sickle cell anemia a molecular disease. Science. 1949;**110**(2865):543-548

[20] Kato GJ, Steinberg MH, Gladwin MT. Intravascular hemolysis and the pathophysiology of sickle cell disease. The Journal of Clinical Investigation. 2017;**127**(3):750-760

[21] Ataga KI, Orringer EP. Renal abnormalities in sickle cell disease. American Journal of Hematology. 2000;**63**(4):205-211

[22] Allon M. Renal abnormalities in sickle cell disease. Archives of Internal Medicine. 1990;**150**(3):501-504

[23] de Jong PE, van Statius Eps LW. Sickle cell nephropathy: New insights into its pathophysiology. Kidney International. 1985;**27**(5):711-717

[24] Alleyne GA. The kidney in sickle cell anemia. Kidney International. 1975;**7**(6):371-379

[25] Buckalew VM Jr, Someren A. Renal manifestations of sickle cell disease. Archives of Internal Medicine. 1974;**133**(4):660-669

[26] Sundd P, Gladwin MT, Novelli EM. Pathophysiology of sickle cell disease. Annual Review of Pathology. 2019;**14**:263-292

[27] Lebensburger JD et al. Prevalence of acute kidney injury during pediatric admissions for acute chest syndrome. Pediatric Nephrology. 2016;**31**(8):1363-1368

[28] Baddam S et al. Acute kidney injury during a pediatric sickle cell vaso-occlusive pain crisis. Pediatric Nephrology. 2017;**32**(8):1451-1456

[29] Hsu CY. Yes, AKI truly leads to CKD. Journal of American Society Nephrology. 2012;**23**(6):967-969

[30] Hsu RK, Hsu CY. The role of acute kidney injury in chronic kidney disease. Seminars in Nephrology. 2016;**36**(4):283-292

[31] Aban I et al. Severe anemia early in life as a risk factor for sickle-cell kidney disease. Blood. 2017;**129**(3):385-387

[32] Chaturvedi S et al. Rapidly progressive acute chest syndrome in individuals with sickle cell anemia: A distinct acute chest syndrome phenotype. American Journal of Hematology. 2016;**91**(12):1185-1190

[33] Reiter CD et al. Cell-free hemoglobin limits nitric oxide bioavailability in sickle-cell disease. Nature Medicine. 2002;**8**(12):1383-1389

[34] Gladwin MT, Kanias T, Kim-Shapiro DB. Hemolysis and cell-free hemoglobin drive an intrinsic mechanism for human disease. The Journal of Clinical Investigation. 2012;**122**(4):1205-1208

[35] Docherty JC et al. Mechanism of action of heme oxygenase. A study of heme degradation to bile pigment by 18O labeling. The Journal of Biological Chemistry. 1984;**259**(21):13066-13069

[36] Belcher JD et al. Heme degradation and vascular injury. Antioxidants & Redox Signaling. 2010;**12**(2):233-248

[37] Muller-Eberhard U et al. Plasma concentrations of hemopexin, haptoglobin and heme in patients with various hemolytic diseases. Blood. 1968;**32**(5):811-815

[38] Wochner RD et al. Hemopexin metabolism in sickle-cell disease, porphyrias and control subjects-effects of heme injection. The New England Journal of Medicine. 1974;**290**(15):822-826

[39] Hebbel RP et al. Accelerated autoxidation and heme loss due to instability of sickle hemoglobin. Proceedings of the National Academy of Sciences of the United States of America. 1988;**85**(1):237-241

[40] Basile DP, Anderson MD, Sutton TA. Pathophysiology of acute kidney injury. Comprehensive Physiology. 2012;**2**(2):1303-1353

[41] Tracz MJ, Alam J, Nath KA. Physiology and pathophysiology of heme: Implications for kidney disease. Journal of American Society Nephrology. 2007;**18**(2):414-420

[42] Zager RA. Rhabdomyolysis and myohemoglobinuric acute renal failure. Kidney International. 1996;**49**(2):314-326

[43] Gliozzi ML et al. Hemoglobin alters vitamin carrier uptake and vitamin D metabolism in proximal tubule cells: Implications for sickle cell disease. American Journal of Physiology: Cell Physiology. 2019;**317**(5):C993-C1000

[44] Ghosh S et al. Extracellular hemin crisis triggers acute chest syndrome in sickle mice. The Journal of Clinical Investigation. 2013;**123**(11):4809-4820

[45] Belcher JD et al. Heme triggers TLR4 signaling leading to endothelial cell activation and vaso-occlusion in murine sickle cell disease. Blood. 2014;**123**(3):377-390

[46] Ofori-Acquah SF et al. Hemopexin deficiency promotes acute kidney injury in sickle cell disease. Blood. 2020;**135**(13):1044-1048

[47] Larsson J, Allhorn M, Kerstrom B. The lipocalin alpha(1)-microglobulin binds heme in different species. Archives of Biochemistry and Biophysics. 2004;**432**(2):196-204

[48] Saraf SL. Heme A1M'ed at the kidney in sickle cell disease. Blood. 2020;**135**(13):979-981

[49] Gosmanova EO et al. Prevalence and progression of chronic kidney disease in adult patients with sickle cell disease. Journal of Investigative Medicine. 2014;**62**(5):804-807

[50] Lebensburger J et al. Protective role of hemoglobin and fetal hemoglobin in early kidney disease for children with sickle cell anemia. American Journal of Hematology. 2011;**86**(5):430-432

[51] Day TG et al. Association between hemolysis and albuminuria in adults with sickle cell anemia. Haematologica. 2012;**97**(2):201-205

[52] Gurkan S et al. Lactate dehydrogenase as a predictor of kidney involvement in patients with sickle cell anemia. Pediatric Nephrology. 2010;**25**(10):2123-2127

[53] Hamideh D et al. Albuminuria correlates with hemolysis and NAG and KIM-1 in patients with sickle cell anemia. Pediatric Nephrology. 2014;**29**(10):1997-2003

[54] McClellan AC et al. High one year mortality in adults with sickle cell disease and end-stage renal disease. British Journal of Haematology. 2012;**159**(3):360-367

[55] Praga M et al. Absence of hypoalbuminemia despite massive proteinuria in focal segmental glomerulosclerosis secondary to hyperfiltration. American Journal of Kidney Diseases. 1999;**33**(1):52-58

[56] Helal I et al. Glomerular hyperfiltration: Definitions, mechanisms and clinical implications. Nature Reviews: Nephrology. 2012;**8**(5):293-300

[57] Vazquez B et al. Hyperfiltration is associated with the development of microalbuminuria in patients with sickle cell anemia. American Journal of Hematology. 2014;**89**(12):1156-1157

[58] Guasch A et al. Glomerular involvement in adults with sickle cell hemoglobinopathies: Prevalence and clinical correlates of progressive renal failure. Journal of American Society Nephrology. 2006;**17**(8):2228-2235

[59] Guasch A et al. Evidence that microdeletions in the alpha globin gene protect against the development of sickle cell glomerulopathy in humans. Journal of American Society Nephrology. 1999;**10**(5):1014-1019

[60] Nebor D et al. Alpha-thalassemia is associated with a decreased occurrence and a delayed age-at-onset of albuminuria in sickle cell anemia patients. Blood Cells, Molecules & Diseases. 2010;**45**(2):154-158

[61] Saraf SL et al. Genetic variants and cell-free hemoglobin processing in sickle cell nephropathy. Haematologica. 2015;**100**(10):1275-1284

[62] Ashley-Koch AE et al. MYH9 and APOL1 are both associated with sickle cell disease nephropathy. British Journal of Haematology. 2011;**155**(3):386-394

[63] Kormann R et al. Roles of APOL1 G1 and G2 variants in sickle cell disease patients: Kidney is the main target. British Journal of Haematology. 2017;**179**(2):323-335

[64] Geard A et al. Clinical and genetic predictors of renal dysfunctions in sickle cell anaemia in Cameroon. British Journal of Haematology. 2017;**178**(4):629-639

[65] Afenyi-Annan A et al. Lack of Duffy antigen expression is associated with organ damage in patients with sickle cell disease. Transfusion. 2008;**48**(5):917-924

[66] Nolan VG et al. Estimated glomerular filtration rate in sickle cell anemia is associated with polymorphisms of bone morphogenetic protein receptor 1B. American Journal of Hematology. 2007;**82**(3):179-184

[67] Kopp JB et al. MYH9 is a major-effect risk gene for focal segmental glomerulosclerosis. Nature Genetics. 2008;**40**(10):1175-1184

[68] Kato GJ et al. Vasculopathy in sickle cell disease: Biology, pathophysiology, genetics, translational medicine, and new research directions. American Journal of Hematology. 2009;**84**(9):618-625

[69] Zhang D et al. Neutrophils, platelets, and inflammatory pathways at the nexus of sickle cell disease pathophysiology. Blood. 2016;**127**(7):801-809

[70] Bissonnette ML et al. Medullary microvascular thrombosis and injury in sickle hemoglobin C disease. Journal of American Society Nephrology. 2016;**27**(5):1300-1304

[71] Lusco MA et al. AJKD atlas of renal pathology: Sickle cell nephropathy. American Journal of Kidney Diseases. 2016;**68**(1):e1-e3

[72] Kida Y, Tchao BN, Yamaguchi I. Peritubular capillary rarefaction: A new therapeutic target in chronic kidney disease. Pediatric Nephrology. 2014;**29**(3):333-342

[73] Ghosh S, Tan F, Ofori-Acquah SF. Spatiotemporal dysfunction of the vascular permeability barrier in transgenic mice with sickle cell disease. Anemia. 2012;**2012**:582018

[74] Wagener FA et al. Heme is a potent inducer of inflammation in mice and is counteracted by heme oxygenase. Blood. 2001;**98**(6):1802-1811

[75] Qiu Y et al. Microvasculature-on-a-chip for the long-term study of endothelial barrier dysfunction and microvascular obstruction in disease. Nature Biomedical Engineering. 2018;**2**:453-463

[76] Singla S et al. Hemin causes lung microvascular endothelial barrier dysfunction by necroptotic cell death. American Journal of Respiratory Cell and Molecular Biology. 2017;**57**(3):307-314

[77] Ataga KI et al. Urinary albumin excretion is associated with pulmonary hypertension in sickle cell disease: Potential role of soluble fms-like tyrosine kinase-1. European Journal of Haematology. 2010;**85**(3):257-263

[78] Heimlich JB et al. Endothelin-1 contributes to the progression of renal injury in sickle cell disease via reactive oxygen species. British Journal of Pharmacology. 2016;**173**(2):386-395

[79] Kasztan M et al. Long-term Endothelin-A receptor antagonism provides robust renal protection in humanized sickle cell disease mice. Journal of American Society Nephrology. 2017;**28**(8):2443-2458

[80] Scheinman JI. Sickle cell disease and the kidney. Nature Clinical Practice: Nephrology. 2009;5(2):78-88

[81] Ehling J et al. Quantitative micro-computed tomography imaging of vascular dysfunction in progressive kidney diseases. Journal of American Society Nephrology. 2016;**27**(2):520-532

[82] Bábíčková J et al. Regardless of etiology, progressive renal disease causes ultrastructural and functional alterations of peritubular capillaries. Kidney International. 2017;**91**(1):70-85

[83] Lindenmeyer MT et al. Interstitial vascular rarefaction and reduced VEGF-A expression in human diabetic nephropathy. Journal of American Society Nephrology. 2007;**18**(6):1765-1776

[84] Graça-Souza AV et al. Neutrophil activation by heme: Implications for inflammatory processes. Blood. 2002;**99**(11):4160-4165

[85] Dutra FF et al. Hemolysis-induced lethality involves inflammasome activation by heme. Proceedings of the National Academy of Sciences of the United States of America. 2014;**111**(39):E4110-E4118

[86] Chen G et al. Heme-induced neutrophil extracellular traps contribute to the pathogenesis of sickle cell disease. Blood. 2014;**123**(24):3818-3827

[87] Ma Y et al. Role of neutrophil extracellular traps and vesicles in regulating vascular endothelial permeability. Frontiers in Immunology. 2019;**10**:1037

[88] Alvarez O et al. Effect of hydroxyurea treatment on renal function parameters: Results from the multi-center placebo-controlled BABY HUG clinical trial for infants with sickle cell anemia. Pediatric Blood & Cancer. 2012;**59**(4):668-674

[89] Quinn CT et al. Losartan for the nephropathy of sickle cell anemia: A phase-2, multicenter trial. American Journal of Hematology. 2017;**92**(9):E520-E528

[90] Cerqueira BA et al. Increased concentrations of IL-18 and uric acid

in sickle cell anemia: Contribution of hemolysis, endothelial activation and the inflammasome. Cytokine. 2011;**56**(2):471-476

[91] Parikh CR et al. Urine IL-18 is an early diagnostic marker for acute kidney injury and predicts mortality in the intensive care unit. Journal of American Society Nephrology. 2005;**16**(10):3046-3052

[92] Shen J et al. NLRP3 inflammasome mediates contrast media-induced acute kidney injury by regulating cell apoptosis. Scientific Reports. 2016;**6**:34682

[93] Nath KA et al. Induction of heme oxygenase is a rapid, protective response in rhabdomyolysis in the rat. The Journal of Clinical Investigation. 1992;**90**(1):267-270

[94] Lever JM et al. Heme Oxygenase-1 in kidney health and disease. Antioxidants & Redox Signaling. 2016;**25**(3):165-183

[95] Ramos S et al. Renal control of disease tolerance to malaria. Proceedings of the National Academy of Sciences of the United States of America. 2019;**116**(12):5681-5686

[96] Rubio-Navarro A et al. Podocytes are new cellular targets of haemoglobin-mediated renal damage. The Journal of Pathology. 2018;**244**(3):296-310

Chapter 5

Hearing Damage Caused by Sickle Cell Disease

Mara Rissatto-Lago

Abstract

Sickle cell disease (SCD) is a multisystem disease associated with episodes of acute illness and progressive organ damage, leading to impairment of several organs. It is characterized by vaso-occlusive processes resulting from local hypoxia, increased number of sickled erythrocytes, and dissemination of occlusion to adjacent tissues. SCD has a chronic inflammatory mechanism that affects several organs and systems, including the auditory system. Hearing loss resulting from SCD includes conductive hearing loss, sensorineural hearing loss, in the central auditory system, in addition to otoneurological symptoms. These findings occur in both the adult and pediatric populations. At the end of this chapter, it is expected that the reader will be able to identify the main damages in the auditory system resulting from sickle cell disease, understand the pathophysiology of the damage generated in hearing, as well as understand the main care needed to monitor the hearing health of this population.

Keywords: sickle cell disease, hearing, adults, children, hearing loss

1. Introduction

Sickle cell disease (SCD) is characterized by vaso-occlusive processes resulting from local hypoxia, increased number of sickled erythrocytes, and spread of occlusion to adjacent tissues [1]. SCD has a chronic inflammatory mechanism that affects several organs and systems, including the audit system [2]. Hearing losses resulting from SCD include conductive hearing loss [3–5], sensorineural hearing loss (SNHL), analyzed by conventional pure tone audiometry (PTA), in addition, otoneurological symptoms such as tinnitus and dizziness (vertigo) occur [6, 7], and damage to the central auditory system [8–10]. Studies exclusively analyzing the sensory structure of hearing through otoacoustic emissions (OAEs) were also carried out [10–14]. However, there are reports in the literature that disorders in the auditory system are associated with cognitive deficits and learning difficulties [15, 16].

The PTA determines the subject's minimum sensitivity auditory analyzing frequency and intensity. Sensory alterations are detected by electrophysiological auditory tests – OAE and neural alterations (auditory nerve and brainstem) by ABR test [17].

The knowledge about hearing damage in SCD contribute to health promotion, and measures can be adopted, as well as the institution of treatments, respecting their individuality, to improve the quality of life.

2. Hearing impairments in sickle cell disease

2.1 Pathophysiology applied to hearing loss in sickle cell disease

Hearing damage in SCD possibly has several pathophysiological mechanisms. Conductive hearing loss resulting from middle ear disorders may be caused by upper airway infections [4]. Adenoid hypertrophy may contribute to otitis media with effusion mechanically due to Eustachian tube obstruction, or functioning as a reservoir for otitis media-causing bacteria [18]. Children with SCD are predisposed to adenoid hypertrophy as a response to their functional asplenia, predisposing infections caused by streptococcus pneumoniae and hemophilus influenzae [19]. The prevalence of adenotonsillar hypertrophy in children with SCD was reported to be 55.3% compared to 30–37.6% in children without the disease [20]. Few data are available on the risk and consequences of otitis media in children with SCD. Taipale et al. [5], analyzing a cohort of 61 children with SCD, found 3% of children with acute otitis media, no cases of chronic otitis media, and only 2% with otitis media with effusion. MacDonald et al [21], in the United States, detected 19 cases of otitis media with effusion in a cohort of 84 children. These data are similar to the healthy population. Stuart and Smith, in 2019, state in their study that although they did not collect the etiology of conductive losses, it can be assumed that they were most caused by otitis media [22].

The physiopathology of SNHL in SCD has not been understood. The known hypothesis refers to the reduction of blood circulation in the auditory system due to the deformed shape of the blood cells, resulting in hypoxia in the structures of the auditory system [23–25]. Histopathological study of the temporal bone of a child SNHL and SCD demonstrated conglomerate of sickled erythrocytes in the circulation of the structures of the auditory system (cochlear stria vascularis) and reduction in the number of outer hair cells compatible with hypoxia [26].

The SNHL in SCD apparently affects high frequencies, which can be explained due to the high consumption of the oxygen of the stria vascularis [27]. Lago et al. [2] demonstrated reduced flow-mediated dilation, with ultrasonographic imaging of the brachial artery, in patients with SCD-homozygous (HbSS) – sickle cell anemia (SCA) with SNHL de displaying the role of vascular endothelium dysfunction in vaso-occlusion in SCD associated with SNHL.

2.2 Characteristics and prevalence of hearing damage associated with sickle cell disease

The hearing loss in SCD presents great variation among different studies. Conductive hearing loss occurs in about 27.5% of children and adolescents [4]. A retrospective study analyzes the prevalence of hearing loss in audiometric data of 128 children and adolescents with SCA. The occurrence of hearing loss ranged from 28.8% to 50.8%, according to the method used (i.e. individual vs. ear-specific; any elevated threshold vs. a three-frequency pure tone average). There are more occurrences of conductive hearing loss than SNHL [22].

The prevalence of SNHL in SCD varies from 3.8% [4] to 66% [28] including adults and children and different genotypes (homozygous (HbSS), heterozygous (HBSC) and, thalassemias). This difference may be linked to factors such as genotype, age group, geographic region, socioeconomic aspects, level of sequelae related to the disease, treatments used, and the cutoff point adopted in the evaluation to identify hearing point adopted. A systematic review and meta-analysis study including 12 studies and a total of 636 SCD patients and 360 controls identified 26.3% of SNHL in adults with SCD [29], including different genotypes. Another systematic review, including 14 studies, with 884 homozygous participants aged between 4 and 56 years, found a prevalence of 20.5%.

As to the characteristics of SNHL in SCD patients, the SNHL can occur in both sexes, in one or both ears and, the severity is predominance in the mild range. Apparently, it initially affects effect higher frequencies (4–8 kHz) followed by the low frequencies (0.25–0.5 kHz). The basal portion is metabolically active, and the structures are the main receptors of acoustic energy from the external environment, and it becomes more sensitive to variations and/or deprivation of oxygen or glucose. Changes in other frequencies suggest that the damage is diffuse in the cochlea [30]. Based on the hypothesis of circulatory changes in the auditory system in SCD, variations in SNHL characteristics could be explained by the duration, distribution, and size of the ischemic process in the circulation of the inner ear [4].

Studies demonstrated that SNHL in SCD patients could occur in different age groups (children, adolescents, and young adults). Most of the studies included samples with a wide age range, which led to inaccurate results regarding prevalence by age group. Studies that included only children and adolescents demonstrated high occurrence [2, 22, 31]. Studies with a broad age range showed a greater prevalence over 30 years of age [8, 32, 33]. And, other two studies [6, 34] described a trend toward worsening with increasing age, suggesting that SNHL is progressive in SCD patients. It might be expected that as patients with SCD grow older, and they will experience repeated crises and show an increased incidence of SNHL.

The characteristics of the SNHL are shown in **Table 1**.

In principle, variables such as the treatment used, and even the model of these studies, may interfere in this relationship, since observational cross-sectional studies do not allow identification of the moment of SNHL installation of hemoglobin and fetal hemoglobin levels. Although SNHL may go unnoticed, there are records of patients who developed a severe/profound degree, requiring intervention with electronic devices such as a cochlear implant to restore hearing [40]. The pediatric population presented, in most studies, the severity of mild/moderate hearing loss, which is often not perceptible for the discernment of the children themselves.

Case studies demonstrate sickle cell crisis directly correlating with sudden and sometimes permanent unilateral or bilateral SNHL presentation [25, 41, 42]. While suffering in the midst of an acute pain crisis, one of these patients also experienced debilitating vestibular dysfunction [42].

Rissatto-Lago et al [7] describe a high occurrence of otoneurological symptoms (vertigo and/or tinnitus) in the pediatric population with SCA 46.4 % and concluded that the presence of sickle cells in vascularization in the labyrinthine artery is capable of compromising the vascularization of the structures responsible for body balance, such as the semicircular canals.

Considering the physiopathology and sensitivity of the inner ear, hidden damage can be present and not yet been detected in PTA. The OAE are sounds of cochlear origin, which can be recorded by a microphone fitted into the ear canal. They are caused by the motion of the cochlea's sensory hair cells as they energetically respond to auditory stimulation.

The OAE test is the fast, noninvasive method to identify subclinical alterations in the cochlea. The transient otoacoustic emissions (TOAEs) responses are the strongest, and therefore, the easiest to detect in the primary auditory frequency band of 1–4 kHz, triggered by broad-spectrum acoustic stimulus as whole and detected in

Study (Author, year, and country)	Number of patients (Sex); Genotype	Age (years)	Hearing loss	Rate of SNHL	Laterality, severity
Al-Dabbous et al. (1996); Saudi Arabia [35]	100 (42F/58M) HbSS	5–40	≥ 25 dB at one or more frequencies	19 (19%)	52.6% unilateral; Severity: 10.5% mild; 63.5% moderate; and 26.3% severe range
Al-Muhaimeed et al. (2000); Saudi Arabia [33]	50 (22F/28M) HbSS	4–45	> 20 dB at two or more frequencies	18 (36%)	72% unilateral; Severity: 73.9% mild; 17.4% moderate; and 8.7% severe
Piltcher et al. (2000); Brazil [6]	28 (15M/13F) HbSS	6–55	> 20 dB at two or more frequencies	6 (21.4%)	Tendency to be bilateral Severity: NR
Onakoya et al. (2002); Nigeria [28]	167(96F/73M) HbSS	15–56	> 25 dB at one or more frequencies	110(66%)	62% bilateral; Severity: 58% mild
Mgbor and Emodi (2004); Nigeria [27]	52 (36M/16 F) HbSS	6–19	> 25 dB at one or more frequencies	7 (13.4%)	100% unilateral; Severity: 100% mild
Aderibigbe et al. (2005); Nigeria [34]	46(21M/25F) HbSS	16–48	> 25 dB (mean of frequencies 0.5, 1, 2, and 4 kHz)	4 (4.3%)	100% unilateral; Severity: 100% mild
Jovanovic-Batman and Hedreville (2006); Guadeloupe (France) [8]	79(36M/43F) HbSS; HbSC	16–50	> 20 dB at two or more frequencies in one or both ears	36(45.56%)	NR laterality Severity: 100% mild
Alabi et al. (2008); Nigeria [4]	80 (45M/35F) HbSS	4–15	> 25 dB at one or more frequencies	3 (3.8%)	100% unilateral; Severity: 100% mild
Samperi et al. (2005); Italy [36]	73 Sex: NR 23 HbSS; 50S-β-thalassemia	7–54	> 25 dB at one or more frequencies	24% (S-β-thalassemia) 30% (HbSS)	71,42% unilateral Severity: 100% mild
Onakoya et al. (2010); Nigeria[32]	43 HbSC	15–65	> 25 dB at one or more frequencies	12 (27.9%)	Severity: mild
Al Jabr (2016); Saudi Arabia [37]	40HbSC, HbSS	20–45	>25 dB at one or more frequencies	9 (22.5%)	6 (15%) bilateral Severity: mild
Lago et al. (2018); Brazil[2]	52HbSS (27M/25F)	6–18	> 20 dB at one or more frequencies	15 (28.8%)	(86.66%) unilateral Severity: 100% mild
Olajuyin et al. (2018); Nigeria [31]	81 Sex: NR	5–17	>25 dB (mean value of frequencies of 0.5, 1, 2 kHz)	23 (28.3%)	Severity: majority mild
Bois et al. (2018); France [3]	61	4–19	>20 dB at the mean value of frequencies of 0.5, 1, and 2 kHz	2 (3.27%)	100% unilateral; Severity: moderate

Study (Author, year, and country)	Number of patients (Sex); Genotype	Age (years)	Hearing loss	Rate of SNHL	Laterality, severity
Sarac et al. (2018); Turkey [38]	45 (20M/25F)	18–45	> 25 dB at the mean value of frequencies of 0.5, 1, and 2 kHz	2 (4.4%)	NR
Towerman et al. (2018); United States [39]	60 (*did not discriminate sex in the HbSS Group)	>22	≥ 25 dB at the mean value of frequencies of 0.5, 1, 2, and 4 kHz	3 (5%)	100% unilateral; Severity: 100%moderate
Stuart and Smith (2019); United States [22]	128	3-14	*Variable	3.1% to 17.1% depending on the calculation method employed	Unilateral or bilateral; Severity: 60.0% slight; 5.7% mild; 28.6% moderate; 1.4% severe; and 4.3% profound
Bomfim et al. (2022); Brazil [16]	31 25HbSS 6HbSC (16M;14F)	8–17	>20 dB at one or more frequency	25.8%	Severity: 100% severity mild

kHz, kilohertz; dB, decibel; HL, hearing loss; M, male; F, female; HbSS, hemoglobin SS; HbSC, hemoglobin SC; NR, Not reported.

Table 1.
Prevalence and characteristics of sensorineural hearing loss in sickle cell disease.

subjects. The distortion product otoacoustic emissions (DPOAEs) responses that are generated by the nonlinear interaction of two pure tones presented simultaneously valuates specific parts of the cochlea and varies from 0.5 to 8 kHz, which are the frequencies in subjects with normal hearing or mild hearing loss detected [43, 44].

Differences in the OAE amplitudes were noted in four of the six studies, with an increase in amplitude being identified in the group with SCA [11–14]. The main studies and characteristics of the OAE are shown in **Table 2**.

The increase in OAE amplitude in SCD suggests early changes in cochlear micromechanics, which may progress to the appearance of SNHL. The increase in amplitude may not be attributed to ear and functional differences in the outer values in the mean evaluated in tympanometry [12]. One hypothesis for the increase in OAE amplitude in SCD would be due to aberrant median olivocochlear neural function; however, this hypothesis was found contrary in a study, which no differences in the mean suppression of TOAE between the groups suppress SCD and healthy participants, indicating normal function of the medial or olivocochlear system [14]. This normality of the medial olivocochlear system was also observed in the study by Rissatto-Lago et al. [10], who identified similar DPOAE amplitudes in participants with SCD and hearing thresholds within normal limits when compared to healthy controls.

The association between increased OAE amplitude in participants with SCD who did not receive hydroxyurea (HU) compared to those treated with HU is evidence for the possibility of premature changes in the cochlear micromechanics of the inflammatory process of SCA. As HU is a drug that reduces the inflammatory process in SCA by reducing the adhesion of erythrocytes and leukocytes to the vascular endothelium, it reduces myelosuppression and vasodilation through the release of nitric oxide [45]. It is possible that the return of OAE amplitudes to a normal level reflects a reduction in the mechanism of the undetermined cause of the increase in OAE amplitude.

Study	Participants Fri; Age (years)	Results
Downs et al. (2000); United States	20 (11M/9F); 6–13	DPOAE amplitudes significantly larger for the SCA group; lower amplitude for the lower frequencies
Walker et al. (2004); United States	12 (5M/7F); 6–14	DPOAE amplitudes were significantly larger for the SCA group; reduced amplitude for lower frequencies
Stuart et al. (2012); United States	30 Group I: 15 treated HDU (9M/6F) Group II: 15 non-treated HDUs (6M/9F)	DPOAE amplitudes were significantly larger in the SCA group not treated with HDU in comparison with the SCA group treated with HDU and the healthy controls; lower amplitude for the lower frequencies
Stuart and Preast (2012); United States	13 (5M/7F) 5–17	TOAE amplitudes were significantly larger for the SCA group. There was no difference in the mean to inhibit evaluating effects of the MOC system (effects suppression) between the groups with SCA and HC.
Kegele et al. (2015); Ghana	35 (Fri NR) 6 months–10 years	There was no difference relative to the presence and amplitude of TOAEs in the comparison between the SCA group and HC
Lake et al. (2018); Brazil	37 (20M/17F); 6–18	There was no statistically significant difference in the DPOAE amplitudes between the SCA and healthy controls groups. No difference in the absolute level of inhibition effects of the MOC between SCA and HC.

F, female sex; M, male sex; DPOAE, distortion product otoacoustic emissions; HDU, hydroxyurea; SCA, sickle cell anemia; TOAE, transient otoacoustic emissions.

Table 2.
Studies with sickle cell disease (homozygous) using the tests of transient and distortion product otoacoustic emissions (n = 6).

The iron chelator deferoxamine, administered parenterally, or deferasirox orally are ototoxic drugs and may cause permanent or transient hearing deficits depending on the dosage and time of exposure to the medication. These ototoxic effects culminate in changes in the cochlea and a reduction in the number of outer hair cells [35].

Damage to the central auditory pathways must be considered, including subclinical damage such as hidden damage to the auditory system. Increased contralateral acoustic reflexes were found in homozygous SCD children and adolescents, with hearing thresholds within normal limits. According to the authors, considering that alterations in the brainstem or efferent system can affect the level of the acoustic reflex in the presence of integrity of the afferent pathway, and the hypothesis of possible retrocochlear alterations (brain stem) is raised. This study auditory brainstem response (ABR) mean latencies of waves III and V and the mean interpeak latencies I–III and IV are significantly higher in the SCD patients, compared to the healthy group [10].

A study in France found changes in the ABR in 25.35% of patients with SCD compared to healthy controls due to an increase in interpeak latencies (III–V), and men were the most affected by this alteration [8]. In another study, Husain et al (2011) reported that 51% of patients with SCD had altered ABR results suggesting damage to a portion of the brainstem (retrocochlear alteration) [9].

P300 is an auditory cognitive evoked potential involved in attention, discrimination, and memory. It is an indicator of cortical processing, speed, and delay in patients with cognitive deterioration [46]. Children with SCD had a longer P300 latency compared to the control group; however, none of the SCD morbidity markers were related to P300 [15]. However, it is still controversial, as another study, including children and adolescents with SCD, found similar P300 responses between patients with SCD and controls [47]. Similar results were found by Rissatto-Lago et al [10], in which children and adolescents with clinically stable SCD had similar P300 latencies with healthy controls.

2.3 Conduct and clinical applicability

Damage to the auditory system in patients with SCD, including the pediatric population, seems quite evident, making it clear that risk detection for hearing disorders should focus on young people, in order to accurately detect subclinical changes that can progress to sensory impairments. SNHL hearing impairments already installed in a very young population is a very relevant fact and requires particular attention from specialists who deal with these patients, considering that, in addition to influencing quality of life, good hearing is crucial for learning and school performance, which can also be harmed by this factor, and a periodic hearing assessment is indicated.

Thus, patients who underwent hearing assessment at birth (neonatal hearing screening) with positive results should be audiologically monitored. Audiological procedures, such as OAE exams, can be ordered at any age, assessing sensory integrity. Patients using ototoxic medications, for example, iron chelator deferoxamine or deferasirox, should be monitored more carefully and in a short period of time.

Hearing assessment, including behavioral procedures such as pure tone audiometry and immitanciometry, should be requested at the beginning of literacy, even for participants without auditory signs or symptoms, since studies have shown that the presence of mild impairments may be associated with school difficulties. And when possible, an evaluation with ABR should be performed to monitor the central auditory pathway in order to detect damage that may manifest with advancing age.

3. Conclusions

There is a higher prevalence of SNHL in patients with SCD compared to the general population. This is likely due to the pathophysiology of the disease and the hematologic effects on the labyrinthine microvasculature. The otorhinolaryngologist must be aware of the otological manifestations of SCD such as SNHL and request periodic assessment of the auditory function of patients with SCD.

Acknowledgements

The author would like to thank professors Ana Marice Teixera Ladeia and Cristina Salles for the teachings and contributions in the works that resulted in the construction of this chapter.

Conflict of interest

The author declares no conflict of interest.

Author details

Mara Rissatto-Lago
Department of the Life Science, College of Speech Therapy, State University of Bahia, Salvador, Brazil

*Address all correspondence to: mararissattolago@gmail.com

References

[1] Serjeant GR. Sickle-cell disease. Lancet. 1997;**350**:725-730

[2] Lago MRR, Fernandes C, Lyra IM, Ramos RT, Teixeira R, Salles C, et al. Sensorineural hearing loss in children with sickle cell anemia and its association with endothelial dysfunction. Hematology. 2018;**23**:849-855. DOI: 10.1080/10245332.2018.1478494

[3] Bois E, Francois M, Benkerrou M, Van Den Abbeele T, Teissier N. Hearing loss in children with sickle cell disease: A prospective French cohort study. Pediatric Blood & Cancer. 2019;**66**:1-6. DOI: 10.1002/pbc.27468

[4] Alabi S, Ernest K, Eletta P, Owolabi A, Afolabi A, Suleiman O. Otological findings among Nigerian children with sickle cell anaemia. International Journal of Pediatric Otorhinolaryngology. 2008;**72**:659-663. DOI: 10.1016/j.ijporl.2008.01.024

[5] Taipale A, Pelkonen T, Bernardino L, Peltola H, Pitkaranta A. Hearing loss in Angolan children with sickle-cell disease. Pediatrics International. 2012;**54**:854-857. DOI: 10.1111/j.1442-200X.2012.03719.x

[6] Piltcher O, Cigana L, Friedriech J, Andrade F De, Ribeiro Q, Selaimen S. Sensorineural hearing loss among sickle cell disease patients from southern Brazil. American Journal of Otolaryngology 2000;21:75-79

[7] Rissatto-Lago MR, Salles C, de Pinho FGC, Menezes Lyra I, Terse-Ramos R, Teixeira R, et al. Association between endothelial dysfunction and otoneurological symptoms in children with sickle cell disease. Hematology. 2017;**22**:299-303. DOI: 10.1080/10245332.2016.1261982

[8] Jovanovic-Bateman L, Hedreville R. Sensorineural hearing loss with brainstem auditory evoked responses changes in homozygote and heterozygote sickle cell patients in Guadeloupe (France). The Journal of Laryngology and Otology. 2006;**120**:627-630. DOI: 10.1017/S0022215106001678

[9] Husain A, Habib SS, Al Drees A, Omar SA, Mujeed AS. Short-latency brainsteim auditory-evoked responses associated with homozigous sickle cell disease. Journal of Applied Hematology. 2011;**2**:197-199. DOI: 10.4103/0256-4947.72265

[10] Rissatto Lago MR, da Cruz Fernandes L, Lyra IM, Terse Ramos R, Teixeira R, Salles C, et al. Hidden hearing loss in children and adolescents with sickle cell anemia. International Journal of Pediatric Otorhinolaryngology. 2019;**116**:186-191. DOI: 10.1016/j.ijporl.2018.10.042

[11] Downs CR, Stuart A, Holbert D. Distortion product otoacoustic emissions in normal-hearing children with homozygous sickle cell disease. Journal of Communication Disorders. 2000;**33**:111-119

[12] Walker LJ, Stuart A, Green WB. Outer and middle ear status and distortion product otoacoustic emissions in children with sickle cell disease. American Journal of Audiology. 2004;**13**:164-172

[13] Stuart A, Jones SM, Walker LJ. Insights into elevated distortion product otoacoustic emissions in sickle cell disease: Comparisons of hydroxyurea-treated and non-treated young children. Hearing Research. 2006;**212**:83-89. DOI: 10.1016/j.heares.2005.10.014

[14] Stuart A, Preast JL. Contralateral suppression of transient-evoked otoacoustic emissions in children with sickle cell disease. Ear and Hearing. 2012;**33**:421-429. DOI: 10.1097/AUD.0b013e31823effd9

[15] Ohanian M, Rozovski U, Ravandi F, Garcia-Manero G, Jabbour E, Kantarjian HM, et al. Cognitive evoked potentials and neural networks are abnormal in children with sickle cell disease and not related to the degree of anaemia, pain and silent infarcts. British Journal of Haematology. 2015;**169**:595-597. DOI: 10.1111/bjh.13230

[16] Raiza Fontes Barros Bomfim J, Orge Anunciação Bacelar C, Marques da Silva Neto M, Salles C, Marice Teixeira Ladeia A, Renata Rissatto-Lago M. Association between hearing impairment, school performance and cognitive function in children and adolescents with sickle cell disease. Tropical Medicine & International Health. 2022:1-7. DOI: 10.1111/tmi.13722

[17] Fernandes LC. Dysfunction of the peripheral and central auditory pathway in patients with type 1 diabetes mellitus. Journal of Diabetes Mellitus. 2012;**02**:76-81. DOI: 10.4236/jdm.2012.21012

[18] Saafan ME, Ibrahim WS, Tomoum MO. Role of adenoid biofilm in chronic otitis media with effusion in children. European Archives of Oto-Rhino-Laryngology. 2013;**270**:2417-2425. DOI: 10.1007/s00405-012-2259-1

[19] Rees DC, Williams TN, Gladwin MT. Sickle-cell disease. Lancet. 2010;**376**:2018-2031. DOI: 10.1016/S0140-6736(10)61029-X

[20] Salles C, Ramos RTT, Daltro C, Nascimento VM, Matos MA. Association between adenotonsillar hypertrophy, tonsillitis and painful crises in sickle cell disease. Jornal de Pediatria. 2009;**85**:249-253. DOI: 10.2223/JPED.1898

[21] MacDonald CB, Bauer PW, Cox LC, McMahon L. Otologic findings in a pediatric cohort with sickle cell disease. International Journal of Pediatric Otorhinolaryngology. 1999;**47**:23-28. DOI: 10.1016/S0165-5876(98)90152-5

[22] Stuart A, Smith MR. The emergence and prevalence of hearing loss in children with homozygous sickle cell disease. International Journal of Pediatric Otorhinolaryngology. 2019;**123**:69-74. DOI: 10.1016/j.ijporl.2019.04.032

[23] Saito N, Nadgir RN, Flower EN, Sakai O. Clinical and radiologic manifestations of sickle cell disease in the head and neck. Radiographics. 2010;**30**:1021-1034. DOI: 10.1148/rg.304095171

[24] Saito N, Watanabe M, Liao J, Flower EN, Nadgir RN, Steinberg MH, et al. Clinical and radiologic findings of inner ear involvement in sickle cell disease. American Journal of Neuroradiology. 2011;**32**:2160-2164. DOI: 10.3174/ajnr.A2720

[25] Whitehead RE, MacDonald CB, Melhem ER, McMahon L. Spontaneous labyrinthine hemorrhage in sickle cell disease. American Journal of Neuroradiology. 1998;**19**:1437-1440

[26] Morgenstein KM, Manace ED. Temporal bone histopathology in sickle cell disease. Laryngoscope. 1969;**79**:2172-2180. DOI: 10.1288/00005537-196912000-00013

[27] Mgbor N, Emodi I. Sensorineural hearing loss in Nigerian children with sickle cell disease. International Journal of Pediatric Otorhinolaryngology. 2004;**68**:1413-1416. DOI: 10.1016/j.ijporl.2004.05.009

[28] Onakoya PA, Nwaorgu OGB, Shokunbi WA. Sensorineural hearing loss in adults with sickle cell anaemia. African Journal of Medicine and Medical Sciences. 2002;**31**:21-24

[29] Kapoor E, Strum D, Shim T, Kim S, Sabetrasekh P, Monfared A. Characterization of sensorineural hearing loss in adult patients with sickle cell disease: A systematic review and meta-analysis. Otology & Neurotology. 2021;**42**:30-37. DOI: 10.1097/MAO.0000000000002825

[30] Rissatto Lago MR, Fernandes LC, Alves G, de Oliveira G, de Andrade O, Salles C, et al. Dysfunction of the auditory system in sickle cell anaemia: A systematic review with meta-analysis. Tropical Medicine & International Health. 2019;**24**:1264-1276. DOI: 10.1111/tmi.13307

[31] Olajuyin OA, Olatunya OS, Adegbiji AW, Oyenibi AS, Faboya OA. Otological burdens of Nigerian children with sickle cell disease. International Journal of Pediatric Otorhinolaryngology. 2018;**107**:1-5. DOI: 10.1016/j.ijporl.2018.01.020

[32] Onakoya PA, Nwaorgu OGB, Shokunbi WA. Hearing impairment in persons with the hemoglobin SC genotype. Ear, Nose, & Throat Journal. 2010;**89**:306-310

[33] Al-Muhaimeed H, Thomas G, Sedran A, Nasher H. Pattern of hearing loss in sickle cell disease. Australian Journal of Oto-Laryngology. 2000;**3**:472-475

[34] Aderibigbe A, Ologe FE, Oyejola BA. Hearing thresholds in sickle cell anemia patients: Emerging new trends? Journal of the National Medical Association. 2005;**97**:1135-1142

[35] Al-Dabbous I, Jam'a AH, Obeja SK, Murugan ANR, Hammad HA. Sensorineural hearing loss in homozygous sickle cell disease in Qatif, Saudi Arabia. Annals of Saudi Medicine. 1996;**16**:641-644

[36] Samperi P, Bertuna G, Rossi G, Poli G, Serra A. Sensorioneural hearing loss in sickle cell disease patientes in Sicily. Minerva Pediatrica. 2005;**57**:285-288

[37] Al Jabr I. Hearing loss among adults with sickle cell disease in an endemic region: A prospective case-control study. Annals of Saudi Medicine. 2016;**36**:135-138

[38] Sarac ET, Boke B, Okuyucu S. Evaluation of hearing and balance functions of patients with sickle cell anemia. Audiology and Neurotology. 2018;**23**:122-125. DOI: 10.1159/000492171

[39] Towerman AS, Hayashi SS, Hayashi RJ, Hulbert ML. Prevalence and nature of hearing loss in a cohort of children with sickle cell disease. Pediatric Blood & Cancer. 2018:1-8. DOI: 10.1002/pbc.27457

[40] Ashfield T, Pai I, Wilson K, Britz A, Connor S, Fitzgerald-O'Connor A, et al. Cochlear implantation in children with sickle cell disease. Pediatrics International. 2015;**57**:174-176. DOI: 10.1111/ped.12413

[41] Orchik DJ, Dunn JW. Sickle cell anemia and sudden deafness. Archives of Otolaryngology. 1977;**103**:369-370

[42] Schreibstein JM, MacDonald CB, Cox LC, McMahon L, Bloom DL. Sudden hearing loss in sickle cell disease: A case report. Otolaryngology and Head and Neck Surgery. 1997;**116**:541-544

[43] Kemp DT. Otoacoustic emissions, their origin in cochlear function, and use. British Medical Bulletin. 2002;**63**:223-241

[44] Kemp DT. Stimulated acoustic emissions from within the human auditory system. The Journal of the Acoustical Society of America. 1978;**64**:1386-1391

[45] Manwani D, Frenette PS. Vaso-occlusion in sickle cell disease: Pathophysiology and novel targeted therapies. Hematology. American Society of Hematology. Education Program. 2013;**2013**:362-369. DOI: 10.1182/asheducation-2013.1.362

[46] Polich J, Kok A. Cognitive and biological determinants of P300: An integrative review. Biological Psychology. 1995;**41**:103-146. DOI: 10.1016/0301-0511(95)05130-9

[47] de Silva IM, Magalhães IQ, Toscano RA, Gandolfi L, Pratesi R. Auditory-evoked response analysis in Brazilian patients with sickle cell disease. International Journal of Audiology. 2010;**49**:272-276. DOI: 10.3109/14992020903321742

Section 2

Sociological Dimension of Sickle Cell Disease

Chapter 6

Role of Sociodemographic and Economic Variables in Predisposition to Vaso-Occlusive Crisis and Mortality in Patients with SCD: Case Study of Sub-Saharan Africa

Osaro Erhabor, Teddy Charles Adias, Tosan Erhabor, Osaro Mgbere, Sadiya Usman and Bibiana Nonye Egenti

Abstract

Sickle cell disease (SCD) is a major public health challenge. It is a common cause of acute and chronic illness and death, which results from a single amino acid substitution (glutamic acid to valine) at position 6 of the beta (β) chain of the hemoglobin molecule. The pathophysiology is based on the polymerization of deoxygenated hemoglobin S (HbS) and production of irreversibly sickled red cells and vaso-occlusive crisis (VOC). The disease is associated with recurrent episodes of acute pain and organ damage. This chapter highlights the role of SES on the predisposition to VOC and mortality among SCD patients. Findings from this review will enable the development and implementation of policies that can facilitate the effective management of SCD in the region. More awareness and education of parents of children and adults living with SCD are needed to identify factors that predispose patients to VOC and common-sense measures to prevent these triggers. SCD patients should be protected against malaria. The need for nutritional intervention, proper hydration, avoidance of dietary intake of sodium, strenuous physical activity, and extreme weather to reduce the incidence of VOC cannot be overemphasized. Protective immunization and access to effective prophylactic and therapeutic agents should be implemented.

Keywords: sociodemography, economy, vaso-occlusive crisis, mortality, SCD, sub-Saharan Africa

1. Introduction

Sickle cell disease (SCD) is of major public health challenge globally, with majority of affected patients residing in sub-Saharan Africa [1]. It is a genetic disorder resulting from the inheritance of abnormal gene (HbS) from both parents [2]. The difference between the abnormal hemoglobin S (HbS) and the normal adult hemoglobin A is a single amino acid substitution of valine for glutamic acid in the sixth position in the β-globin chain. In sub-Saharan Africa, about 300,000 infants are born with major hemoglobin disorders and about 2% of all children have SCD [3]. The frequency of the trait is between 15 and 30% in West Africa [4]. SCD disproportionately affects people in the African continent compared to other parts of the globe. The United Nations estimates that 12–15 million of the world's 25 million SCD patients live in the African continent [5], while an insignificant 10% live in high-income countries (HICs) [6]. The mortality rate from the disease in children under 5 years of age is estimated to exceed 50% in the African continent where healthcare infrastructure is suboptimal and the population are significantly impoverished [7]. Recurrent and random episodes of vaso-occlusive crisis (VOC) are the hallmark of sickle cell disease. The pathophysiology of vaso-occlusive crisis lies in the fact that upon deoxygenation, the mutant HbS molecule polymerizes and attains a characteristic sickle shape. The sickle-shaped red cells adhere to leukocytes immobilized to the endothelium, causing microvascular occlusion and vaso-occlusive crisis (VOC), tissue ischemia, and resultant pain. The actual causes of VOC are unknown. However, factors including exposure to cold (hypothermal), dehydration, infection, malaria infection, and stress may play a role [8]. Painful vaso-occlusive crisis (VOC) is the commonest cause of hospital admission in patients with SCD. Socioeconomic status (SES) and demographic variables seem to play a key role in the prevalence, development of complications, and mortality in several diseases including sickle cell disease (SCD) and particularly in low-income developing countries. The aim of this chapter is to review the several sociodemographic and socioeconomic variables that can predispose to vaso-occlusive crisis among sickle cell disease patients.

2. Effects of sociodemographic and economic factors in VOC in SCD

Sociodemographic variables play a role in hospitalization of SCA children. The level of educational attainment of parents has a significant role in the incidence and presentation to hospital with VOC. A previous report in Sokoto, North Western Nigeria, indicated that majority of the parents of children presenting to the children emergency unit with vaso-occlusive crisis were either educated up to secondary school or had no formal education. Also, a SCD child's position in a family had a role in presentation in emergency unit with VOC. Majority of the subject presenting to hospital in VOC were $\geq$ 6th position [9]. Higher levels of education and income mitigate the deleterious effects of the psychosocial consequences (anxiety and depression) associated with SCD. Parents of SCD children with higher education or income are more likely to make better informed decision about nutritional requirements and use of insecticide-treated mosquito nets to protect their children from malaria. They are also able to afford the medication and the various treatment options required for the effective management of their SCD children [10]. There are several factors that play a role in an individual's socioeconomic status (education, profession, and income). SES of an individual can play a role in the development, complications, negative outcome, and increased mortality of patients with SCD [11]. The effects of these factors often begin in the prenatal stages before a child is born and tend to continue through life [12]. A study that investigated the influence of SES factors on hematological and clinical parameters in children with SCD in Saudi Arabia [13] indicated that a significant number of children affected with the SCD were from the low socioeconomic class on <5000 SAR. The prevalence of VOC, adverse events, and more deranged hematological indices was more prevalent among patients in the lowest SES.

2.1 Role of poverty on incidence of VOD in SCD patients

Inability to pay for healthcare can have a significant effect on accessibility and promptness of assessing care for many indigent patients. Many SCD patients do not access care on time until complications have developed. This can potentially result in longer lengths of stay for the treatment of complications of their underlying disease [14]. A previous report in Sokoto, North Western Nigeria, indicated that majority of the parents of children in vaso-occlusive crisis had income of < N36,000 naira (equivalent of <$75) monthly [9]. The management of SCD patients is not cheap. In the United States, the estimated total healthcare cost per year for children and adults with SCD stand at USD1.1 billion [15]. Children from low socioeconomic status (SES) with and without chronic disease have been reported to have worse health outcomes and higher utilization of health resources compared to those who are more advantaged [16]. They are more likely to be admitted to the hospital, have longer lengths of hospital stay, and generate more healthcare-associated costs particularly in the first 10 years of life compared to children from higher SES [17]. However, a previous report that examined the association between socioeconomic status and length of hospital stay for children with sickle cell disease observed that SES has no clinically important effect on the length of hospital stay [18]. Efforts are being made to better understand the pathophysiology, prevent and ameliorate the consequences, and ensure the effective management of VOC in sickle cell disease using novel targeted therapies [19]. The major challenge that may limit the access to these therapies in developing countries where this disease is more prevalent is cost [20]. Managing patients with SCD comes with a huge cost [21]. In 2004 alone, more than 80,000 hospitalizations were attributable to adult SCD patients in the United States, costing nearly $500 million, with majority of the cost arising from inpatient hospitalization associated with VOC [8, 22]. Managing chronic illness like SCD in low- and middle-income countries (LMICs) can incur very high out-of-pocket (OOP) payments for healthcare. Many households do not have the necessary money. Some are left with no other option than to adopt one or more "coping strategies," such as borrowing money often times at outrageous interest rates, or selling assets like land, farm produce, and jewelleries [23]. Out-of-pocket expenditure can prevent a number of SCDs from accessing care promptly due to unaffordability, and this can affect the delivery of a prompt and efficient management of patients with sickle cell disease [24]. There is need for government across sub-Saharan Africa to provide universal access to quality care for patients with SCD as well as to improve the awareness among patients on the need to promptly access care to prevent complications. These implementations can potentially help improve health outcomes.

2.2 Effect of malnutrition on the incidence of VOC in SCD

There seems an interconnection between nutritional state, host defense, susceptibility, and disease outcomes. Previous report indicates that micronutrient deficiencies are associated with signs of poor growth, increased susceptibility to infection, and recurrent occurrences of VOC in patients with SCD and outcomes [25].

The important role nutrition plays in the health-related quality of life of patients cannot be overemphasized. A previous report indicated that the health-related quality of life of a cohort of SCD patients improved significantly after tailored micronutrient program was initiated among the patients [26, 27]. Qualitative malnutrition seen among SCD tends to be multifactorial and often results from suboptimal intake or uptake of macro- or micronutrients. SCD-related increased nutritional demands, presence of attendant chronic gastrointestinal diseases and infections, socioeconomic status, and lifestyle factors tend to predispose SCD patients to frequent hospitalizations primarily due to vaso-occlusive crises and other SCD-related complications [28]. Zinc and omega-3 fatty acid supplementation have been associated with limited reduction in vaso-occlusive crises [29]. The disparity in SES, migrations, food insecurity, fast-food habits, and social and cultural patterns seem to be the main causes of altered nutrition in individuals throughout the globe [30]. Suboptimal intake of macro- and micronutrients has been shown to be associated with predisposition and negative outcomes in SCD patients. Micronutrient deficiencies, including zinc, copper, folic acid, pyridoxine, vitamin E, B_6, and B_{12}, omega-3 fatty acids, vitamin D, and arginine have been shown to play a role [31–34]. Similarly, the use L-glutamine has been shown to be beneficial in decreasing the incidents of SCD-related vaso-occlusive (VOC) pain events without significant safety concerns [35]. Zinc supplementation has been associated with decreased incidence of infections, number of hospitalizations, and vaso-occlusive pain crisis among SCD patients [36]. The serum copper, selenium, RBC, HCT, HGB, MCV, MCH, and MCHC were significantly lower among sickle cell disease patients compared to controls. It is recommended that trace elements (copper and selenium) and hematological parameters are monitored routinely among sickle cell disease children to optimize the care offered to these individuals [9]. Vaso-occlusion is understood to be the root cause of sickle cell pain. Nitric oxide (NO) is a potent vasodilator [37] that plays a role in the vaso-occlusive complications of SCD [38]. Recent findings indicate that one of the pathophysiological pathways of sickle cell disease (SCD) lies on the role of red cell hemolysis and nitric oxide (NO) depletion on the occurrence of acute and chronic complications including VOC. Nitric oxide is produced in the endothelium from its obligate substrate L-arginine, which is converted to citrulline by a family of enzymes, the NO synthases (NOS). *P. falciparum* malaria is a common trigger of VOC in SCD patients. *P. falciparum* malaria is associated with hypoarginaemia among preschool children of African descent [39]. Arginine is a safe and inexpensive intervention with narcotic-sparing effects that may be a beneficial adjunct to standard therapy for sickle-cell-related pain in children [40–42]. SCD children have lower values of antioxidant enzymes compared to controls. Superoxide dismutase (SOD) and glutathione peroxidase (GPX) levels in sickle cell disease patient in vaso-occlusive crisis are significantly lower compared to that of non-sickle cell controls [43]. There seems a justification to urgently develop dietary reference intakes (DRIs) and recommended dietary allowances (RDAs) for patients with SCD and integrate nutritional intervention as a vital adjunct in the prevention of VOC and the treatment of patients [44].

2.3 Socioeconomic disparity in access to health

SES is defined as a complex combination of several factors including occupation, income, knowledge, education, and power in a society that affect an individual's well-being [45]. The quality of healthcare delivery is on a decline in many developing economies and limits access to health products particularly for those with low

SES [46]. Abnormal growth, stunting, and a low BMI are commoner in children with SCD of lower socioeconomic class [47]. Data from the United Kingdom shows that SCD children from low SES constitutes the majority of those hospitalized. The hospital admissions were majorly due to episodes of VOC [18]. The need for government particularly in low-income settings to address the issue of inequalities in access to health products cannot be overemphasized. There is disparity in access to care in SCD in urban setting compared to those in rural settings. Reports from the island of Jamaica and the United States indicate that SCD patients with more severe genotypes tend to live in higher poverty-stricken rural settings and tend to travel longer distance to access healthcare services and advocate that government particularly in developing countries ensure that better access to healthcare services is provided for SCD patients residing in rural settings [48–50].

2.4 Lack of education and awareness on the management of patients at home to prevent the risk of VOC

Painful crises are the causes of 50–60% of emergency visits and 60–80% of hospitalizations in children with SCD [51]. Triggers for VOC vary and can include inflammation, stress, increased viscosity, decreased flow, hemolysis, infection, exposure to cold, hypoxia, acidosis, dehydration, physically demanding activity, emotional stress, and malaria, or a combination of factors [19, 52]. A previous report from Nigeria indicates that malaria (76.7%) and bacterial infection (60%) were common trigger of VOC among SCD subjects [9]. A significant association has been observed between the parents' awareness of VOCs and a better disease outcome in their children, as they had fewer attacks and hospital admissions [53]. The need to provide information required to enable parents of children and adults with SCD effectively manage themselves at home to reduce the incidence VOC and need for hospitalization cannot be overemphasized. There are a number of commonsense measures that can be implemented to reduce the risk of VOC-related admissions. Parents of children and adult patients with SCD must take the issue of optimal hydration seriously. Poorly hydrated erythrocytes lead to increased viscosity and may contribute to the vaso-occlusive crisis in SCD [54]. It is crucial for SCD patients to promote proper hydration by frequent intake of water, avoidance of dietary intake of sodium, and avoidance of strenuous physical activity and extreme weather that result in excessive sweating [55, 56]. Majority of SCD patients live in *Plasmodium falciparum* endemic African countries [57]. SCD patients are highly vulnerable to malaria infection as a result of impaired splenic function which is a common feature in SCD patients [58]. Infection with *Plasmodium falciparum* in SCD patients can trigger painful vaso-occlusive crisis, increase the severity of anemia, and contribute to early childhood mortality [59]. Efforts must be made to keep SCD patients safe from malaria infection by providing them with antimalarial chemoprophylaxis and insecticides-treated mosquito nets, and the implementation of vector control measures [60, 61]. Evidence from the UK indicates that environmental factors including increased wind speed and low humidity have a significant effect on acute pain in SCD. Others indicates that low levels of carbon monoxide and nitric oxide were associated with increased numbers of VOC-related hospital admissions [62, 63]. Parents of children with SCD and adult patients have a duty of care to ensure that these preventive measures are implemented. Sickle cell disease (SCD) is characterized by recurrent vaso-occlusive crisis (VOC). Patients with SCD tend to have impaired immunity due to splenic infarction which predisposes them to recurrent infections [64]. Other infection predisposing factors in SCD include abnormalities of opsonization, suboptimal antibody production, impaired leukocyte functions, and cell-mediated immunity [65]. The clinical course of the disease is characterized by periodically painful vaso-occlusive crisis, which can be triggered by psychological, physical, and infective factors [66]. Hyposplenism predisposes SCD patients to severe infections with malaria and encapsulated organisms, including *Haemophilus influenza, Mycoplasma pneumoniae, Salmonella typhimurium, Staphylococcus aureus, Escherichia coli, and Streptococcus pneumoniae* [64, 67]. Respiratory tract infections are common in SCD and vary and range from mild upper tract infection to moderately severe uncomplicated pneumonia that can be managed with appropriate antibiotics. Respiratory tract infection if poorly managed can predispose patients to acute chest syndrome (ACS) which is a serious and potentially fatal complication. There is the need to reduce the burden of infection on SCD patients by ensuring that patients are administered the relevant protective immunization, have access to effective prophylactic and therapeutic use of antimicrobial, keep their environment, clean and are provided with barrier protection [68]. There is need for governments across the sub-Saharan Africa to take realistic steps to eradicate poverty and illiteracy as enshrined in the United Nations' millennium development goals for underdeveloped countries. This will go a long way in reducing the high incidence of infection among SCD patients in particular and improving the quality of life of patients.

2.5 Psychosocial realities of vaso-occlusive crisis in SCD

A previous report indicated that sociodemographic characteristics and quality of life play a major role in SCD, and these have serious psychosocial consequences, especially anxiety and depression, on SCD patients [69]. Vaso-occlusive pain crises (VOC) is the most common cause of emergency department visits and hospitalizations in patients with sickle cell disease [70]. Sickle cell disease (SCD) patients with VOC may experience a broad range of mental health disorders. Pediatric patients with SCD and a history of a mental health diagnosis have longer length of stay (LOS) and higher admission rates for the management of VOC. Ultimately, these findings suggest that mental health pose a challenge to the management of VOC-related pain in patients with SCD [71]. Pediatric patients diagnosed with a psychiatric disorder, specifically mood or anxiety disorders, have longer LOS for VOC. These findings suggest that future interventions aimed at managing VOC may need to consider adjunctive psychiatric assessment and intervention [72]. Comorbid depression is significantly associated with longer LOS, more severity of illness, and higher hospital charges [73]. Healthcare providers caring for adults with SCD should consider screening and managing the mental health of SCD patients to improve the health-related quality of life. SCD patients with depression had a higher prevalence of acute vaso-occlusive pain and acute chest syndrome visits per year, developed more complications related to organ damage, and incurred significantly higher outpatient and inpatient total healthcare costs compared to controls [74]. VOC-related acute pain and fatigues resulting from anemia are major hallmarks of SCD. These factors predispose patients to psychological disorders, depression, anxiety, and a negative impact on their quality of life (QoL) [75]. Previous report indicates that the rates of depression in SCD patients (18–46%) are similar to those seen in other chronic diseases [76]. Depression seems prevalent in patients with SCD and may be correlated with demographic and social factors. A previous study investigated the prevalence of depression and anxiety among SCD patients from different sociodemographic groups in Jeddah, Saudi Arabia.

Finding indicated that there was a significant association between depression rate and the two variables of patient employment status (49.3%; p = 0.047) and a family history of SCD (51%) [77]. A depression rate of 48.2% was reported among the SCD patients in Qitaf, Eastern Province of Saudi Arabia [78]. Depression among SCD patients in sub-Saharan African may even be higher for a number of reasons; apart from the fatigue and VOC-associated pain, many SCD patients have to grapple with paying for their healthcare cost which tends to be funded out of pocket, and patients also worry about the availability of safe blood transfusion (lack of effective screening for TTIs, risk of possible hemolytic transfusion reaction, and alloimmunization to foreign donor red cells antigens). Many blood transfusion laboratories in sub-Saharan African countries lack facilities for routine alloantibody screening and extended red cell phenotyping. There is also the risk of iron overload and the cost implication of iron chelation therapy [79]. There are a number of factors that may be responsible for the increased incidence of depression among patients with SCD particularly in low-income settings in sub-Saharan Africa; the higher the rate of healthcare utilization, there are higher costs of out-of-pocket medical care and the challenge associated with the effect of the VOC crisis-related pain [80, 81]. There is need to routinely examine the health-related quality of life and mental health status of SCD in relation to VOC-related pain during hospital admissions and target appropriate psychological interventions for the effective management of pain in these patients [82].

3. Conclusion

This review indicates that socioeconomic and demographic factors play a key role in the prevalence of VOC, development of complications, and mortality in sickle cell disease (SCD) particularly in low-income developing countries.

4. Recommendations

1. Governments across sub-Saharan Africa need to take realistic steps to eradicate poverty and illiteracy as enshrined in the United Nations' millennium development goals for underdeveloped countries. This will go a long way in reducing the high incidence of VOC among SCD and improving the quality of life of patients.

2. There in need for more awareness and education of parents of children and adult living with SCD on the factors that predispose patients to VOC and common-sense measures that can be taken to prevent these triggers.

3. There is need to invest significantly on tackling Goal 10 of the Sustainable Development Goals (SDGs) with the hope of *reducing the growing inequalities and closing the widening inequality in access to SCD-related care as well as* relative income inequality *within and among countries.*

4. Efforts must be made by government of sub-Saharan African countries to keep SCD patient safe from malaria infection by providing them with antimalarial chemoprophylaxis, insecticides-treated mosquito nets, and implementation of vector control measures.

5. SCD patients should be encouraged to ensure proper hydration by frequent intake of water, avoidance of dietary intake of sodium, and avoidance of strenuous physical activity and extreme weather that result in excessive sweating to reduce the incidence of VOC.

6. There seems a justification to urgently develop dietary reference intakes (DRIs) and recommended dietary allowances (RDAs) for patients with SCD and integrate nutritional intervention as a vital adjunct in the prevention of VOC and the treatment of patients.

7. There is the need to reduce the burden of infection on SCD patients by ensuring that patients are administered the relevant protective immunization, have access to effective prophylactic and therapeutic use of antimicrobial, keep their environment clean, and are provided with barrier protection.

8. Government of sub-Saharan African countries should ensure that there is improved access to healthcare services for SCD patients particularly those residing in rural settings.

9. There is need to routinely examine the health-related quality of life, mental health status of SCD in relation to VOC-related pain during hospital admissions and target appropriate psychological interventions for the effective management of pain in these patients.

Author details

Osaro Erhabor[1*], Teddy Charles Adias[2], Tosan Erhabor[3], Osaro Mgbere[4], Sadiya Usman[1] and Bibiana Nonye Egenti[5]

1 Department of Haematology, Usmanu Danfodiyo University Sokoto, Nigeria

2 Federal University Otuoke Bayelsa State, Nigeria

3 Medical Laboratory Science Council of Nigeria, Nigeria

4 Houston Health Department, Disease Prevention and Control Division, Houston, Texas, USA

5 Department of Community Medicine, College of Health Sciences, University of Abuja, Nigeria

*Address all correspondence to: n_osaro@yahoo.com; erhabor.osaro@udusok.edu.ng

References

[1] Rees DC, Williams TN, Gladwin MT. Sickle-cell disease. Lancet. 2010;**376**: 2018-2031. DOI: 10.1016/S0140-6736(10)61029-X

[2] Oniyangi O, Omari AA. Malaria chemoprophylaxis in sickle cell disease. Cochrane Database of Systematic Reviews. 2006;**4**:CD003489

[3] WHO. Sickle-cell Anaemia. Geneva: Author; 2006

[4] Kyerewaa EA, Edwin F, Etwire V. Controlling sickle cell disease in Ghana—ethics and options. The Pan African Medical Journal. 2011;**10**:14

[5] Aliyu ZY, Kato GJ, Taylor JT, Babadoko A, Mamman AI, Gordeuk VR, et al. Sickle cell disease and pulmonary hypertension in Africa: A global perspective and review of epidemiology, pathophysiology, and management. American Journal of Hematology. 2008;**83**:63-70. DOI: 10.1002/ajh.21057

[6] Aygun B, Odame IA. Global perspective on sickle cell disease. Pediatric Blood & Cancer. 2012;**59**:386-390. DOI: 10.1002/pbc.24175

[7] Makani J, Cox SE, Soka D, Komba AN, Oruo J, Mwamtemi H, et al. Mortality in sickle cell anemia in Africa: A prospective cohort study in Tanzania. PLoS One. 2011;**6**:e14699. DOI: 10.1371/journal.pone.0014699

[8] Jang T, Poplawska M, Cimpeanu E, et al. Vaso-occlusive crisis in sickle cell disease: A vicious cycle of secondary events. Journal of Translational Medicine. 2021;**19**:397. DOI: 10.1186/s12967-021-03074-z

[9] Erhabor O, Ogar K, Erhabor T, Dangana A. Some haematological parameters, copper and selenium level among children of African descent with sickle cell disease in Specialist Hospital Sokoto, Nigeria. Human Antibodies. 2019;**27**(3):143-154. DOI: 10.3233/HAB-180360

[10] Ogunfowora OB, Durotoye MO, Gregory AS. A comparative study of academic achievement of children with sickle cell anemia and their healthy siblings. Nigerian Journal of Medicine. 2005;**97**:405-410

[11] Lubeck D, Agodoa I, Bhakta N, Danese M, Pappu K, Howard R, et al. Estimated life expectancy and income of patients with sickle cell disease compared with those without sickle cell disease. JAMA Network Open. 2019;**2**(11):e1915374. DOI: 10.1001/jamanetworkopen.2019.15374

[12] National Research Council Panel on Race, E., Health in Later, L. The National Academies Collection: Reports funded by National Institutes of Health. In: Bulatao RA, Anderson NB, editors. Understanding Racial and Ethnic Differences in Health in Late Life: A Research Agenda. Washington, DC: National Academies Press (US), National Academies; 2004

[13] Khan SA, AlSiny F, Makki A, Ali A, AlAnsari I, Khan S. Socioeconomic status dependent medical complexities in children with sickle cell disease in Saudi Arabia. Saudi Journal of Biological Sciences. 2020;**27**(7):1781-1787. DOI: 10.1016/j.sjbs.2020.03.008

[14] Epstien AM, Stern RS, Weissman JS. Do the poor cost more? A multi-hospital study of patients' socioeconomic status and use of hospital resources. The New England Journal of Medicine. 1991;**322**(16):1122-1128

[15] Kauf TL, Coates TD, Huazhi L, Mody-Patel N, Hartzema AG. The cost of health care for children and adults with sickle cell disease. American Journal of Hematology. 2009;**84**(6):323-327

[16] O'Connor G, Quinton HB, Kneeland T, et al. Median household income and mortality rate in cystic fibrosis. Pediatrics. 2003;**11**(4):333-339

[17] Petrou S, Kupek E. Socioeconomic differences in childhood hospital inpatient service utilization and costs: Prospective cohort study. Journal of Epidemiology and Community Health. 2005;**59**:591-597

[18] Ellison AM, Bauchner H. Socioeconomic status and length of hospital stay in children with vaso-occlusive crises of sickle cell disease. Journal of the National Medical Association. 2007;**99**(3):192-196

[19] Manwani D, Frenette PS. Vaso-occlusion in sickle cell disease: Pathophysiology and novel targeted therapies. Blood. 2013;**122**(24):3892-3898. DOI: 10.1182/blood-2013-05-498311

[20] Telen MJ. Beyond hydroxyurea: New and old drugs in the pipeline for sickle cell disease. Blood. 2016;**127**(7):810-819. DOI: 10.1182/blood-2015-09-618553

[21] Steiner CA, Miller JL. Sickle Cell Disease Patients in U.S. Hospitals, 2004. Rockville, MD: Healthcare Cost and Utilization Project (HCUP) Statistical Briefs; 2006

[22] Brousseau DC, Owens PL, Mosso AL, Panepinto JA, Steiner CA. Acute care utilization and rehospitalizations for sickle cell disease. JAMA. 2010;**303**:1288-1294

[23] Murphy A, McGowan C, McKee M, et al. Coping with healthcare costs for chronic illness in low-income and middle-income countries: A systematic literature review. BMJ Globalization and Health. 2019;**4**:e001475

[24] Ogamba CF, Akinsete AM, Mbaso HS, Adesina OA. Health insurance and the financial implications of sickle cell disease among parents of affected children attending a tertiary facility in Lagos, south-west Nigeria. The Pan African Medical Journal. 2020;**36**:227

[25] Datta D, Namazzi R, Conroy AL, Cusick SE, Hume HA, Tagoola A, et al. Zinc for Infection Prevention in Sickle Cell Anemia (ZIPS): Study protocol for a randomized placebo-controlled trial in Ugandan children with sickle cell anemia. Trials. 2019;**20**(1):460. DOI: 10.1186/s13063-019-3569-z, 20, 1

[26] Martyres DJ, Vijenthira A, Barrowman N, Harris-Janz S, Chretien C, Klaassen RJ. Nutrient insufficiencies/deficiencies in children with sickle cell disease and its association with increased disease severity. Pediatric Blood & Cancer. 2016;**63**(6):1060-1064

[27] Mandese V, Marotti F, Bedetti L, Bigi E, Palazzi G, Iughetti L. Effects of nutritional intake on disease severity in children with sickle cell disease. Nutrition Journal. 2016;**15**(1):46

[28] Ruiz AJ, Buitrago G, Rodríguez N, Gómez G, Sulo S, Gómez C, et al. Clinical and economic outcomes associated with malnutrition in hospitalized patients. Clinical Nutrition. 2019;**38**(3):1310-1316

[29] Dekker LH, Fijnvandraat K, Brabin BJ, van Hensbroek MB. Micronutrients and sickle cell disease, effects on growth, infection and vaso-occlusive crisis: A systematic review. Pediatric Blood & Cancer. 2012;**59**(2):211-215

[30] Cannas G, Merazga S, Virot E. Sickle cell disease and infections in high- and

low-income countries. Mediterranean Journal of Hematology and Infectious Diseases. 2019;**11**(1). DOI: 10.4084/mjhid.2019.042

[31] Hyacinth HI. Sickle-cell anaemia needs more food? Lancet Haematol. 2018;**5**(4):e130. DOI: 10.1016/S2352-3026(18)30032-2

[32] Daak A, Rabinowicz A, Ghebremeskel K. Omega three fatty acids are a potential therapy for patients with sickle cell disease. Nature Reviews. Disease Primers. 2018;**4**:15. DOI: 10.1038/s41572-018-0012-9

[33] Adegoke SA, Smith OS, Adekile AD, ueiredo MS. Relationship between serum 25-hydroxyvitamin D and inflammatory cytokines in paediatric sickle cell disease. Cytokine. 2017;**96**:87-93. DOI: 10.1016/j.cyto.2017.03.010

[34] Morris CR. Alterations of the arginine metabolome in sickle cell disease. A growing rationale for arginine therapy. Hematology/oncology Clinics of North America. 2014;**28**:301-321. DOI: 10.1016/j.hoc.2013.11.008

[35] Quinn CT. L-gutamine for sickle cell anemia: More questions than answers. Blood. 2018;**132**(7):689. DOI: 10.1182/blood-2018-03-834440

[36] Prasad AS, Beck FW, Kaplan J, Chandrasekar PH, Ortega J, et al. Effect of zinc supplementation on incidence of infections and hospital admissions in sickle cell disease (SCD). American Journal of Hematology. 1999;**61**:194-202

[37] Moncada S, Higgs A. The L-arginine-nitric oxide pathway. The New England Journal of Medicine. 1993;**329**(27):2002-2012

[38] Kaul DK, Liu XD, Fabry ME, Nagel RL. Impaired nitric oxide-mediated vasodilation in transgenic sickle mouse. American Journal of Physiology. Heart and Circulatory Physiology. 2000;**278**(6):H1799-H1806

[39] Kabiru M, Erhabor O, Isaac Z, Jiya NM, Knox VD, Abdulrahaman Y, et al. Hypoarginaemia among Pre-School Children of African Descent with Plasmodium Falciparum Malaria. Haematology International Journal. 2017;**1**(1):000102. DOI: 10.23880/HIJ-16000102

[40] Morris CR, Kuypers FA, Lavrisha L, Ansari M, Sweeters N, Stewart M, et al. A randomized, placebo-controlled trial of arginine therapy for the treatment of children with sickle cell disease hospitalized with vaso-occlusive pain episodes. Haematologica. 2013;**98**(9):1375-1382. DOI: 10.3324/haematol.2013.086637

[41] Aslan M, Ryan T, Adler B, Townes T, Parks D, Thompson J, et al. Oxygen radical inhibition of nitric oxide-dependent vascular function in sickle cell disease. Proceedings of the National Academy of Sciences. 2001;**98**(26):15215-15220

[42] Matte A, Cappellini MD, Iolascon A, Enrica F, De Franceschi L. Emerging drugs in randomized controlled trials for sickle cell disease: Are we on the brink of a new era in research and treatment? Expert Opinion on Investigational Drugs. 2020;**29**(1):23-31

[43] Erhabor O, Jiya N, Abubakar M, Usman S. Some antioxidant enzymes among children with sickle cell disease attending Usmanu Danfodiyo University Teaching Hospital Sokoto, North Western Nigeria. Open Journal of Blood Diseases. 2019;**9**:60-76. DOI: 10.4236/ojbd.2019.93007

[44] Umeakunne K, Hibbert JM. Nutrition in sickle cell disease: Recent

insights. Nutrition and Dietary Supplements. 2019;**11**:9-17

[45] Burton DC, Flannery B, Bennett NM, Farley MM, Gershman K, Harrison LH, et al. Active Bacterial Core Surveillance/Emerging Infections Program N. Socioeconomic and racial/ethnic disparities in the incidence of bacteremic pneumonia among US adults. American Journal of Public Health. 2010;**100**:1904-1911

[46] Link-Gelles R, Westreich D, Aiello AE, Shang N, Weber DJ, Holtzman C, et al. Bias with respect to socioeconomic status: A closer look at zip code matching in a pneumococcal vaccine effectiveness study. SSM Population Health. 2016;**2**:587-594

[47] Shah N, Bhor M, Xie L, Halloway R, Arcona S, Paulose J, et al. Treatment patterns and economic burden of sickle-cell disease patients prescribed hydroxyurea: A retrospective claims-based study. Health and Quality of Life Outcomes. 2019;**17**(1):155

[48] Asnani MR, Knight Madden J, Reid M, Greene L-G, Lyew-Ayee P. Socio-environmental exposures and health outcomes among persons with sickle cell disease. PLoS One. 2017;**12**(4):e0175260. DOI: 10.1371/journal.pone.0175260

[49] Haque A, Telfair J. Socioeconomic distress and health status: The urban-rural dichotomy of services utilization for people with sickle cell disorder in North Carolina. The Journal of Rural Health. 2000;**16**:43-55

[50] Telfair J, Haque A, Etienne M, Tang S, Strasser S. Rural/urban differences in access to and utilization of services among people in Alabama with sickle cell disease. Public Health Reports. 2003;**118**:27-36

[51] Meier ER, Miller JL. Sickle cell disease in children. Drugs. 2012;**72**(7):895-906

[52] Yale SH, Guthrie T. Approach to the vaso-occlusive crisis in adults with sickle cell disease. American Family Physician. 2000;**61**(5):1349-1357

[53] Zolaly M, Al-Mohammadi G, Al-Saadi G, Qasim D. Vaso-occlusive crises in patients with sickle cell disease: Parents' perspectives and association with disease outcomes. Journal of Taibah University Medical Sciences. 2019;**14**(6):515-522

[54] Rinehart J, Gulcicek EE, Joiner CH, Lifton RP, Gallagher PG. Determinants of erythrocyte hydration: Current opinion in haematology. Current Opinion in Hematology. 2010;**17**(3):191-197. DOI: 10.1097/MOH.0b013e32833800d0

[55] Diaw M, Samb A, Diop S, et al. Effects of hydration and water deprivation on blood viscosity during a soccer game in sickle cell trait carriers. British Journal of Sports Medicine. 2014;**48**(4):326-331. DOI: 10.1136/bjsports-2012-091038

[56] Williams-Hooker R, Hankins J, Ringwald-Smith K, et al. Evaluation of hydration status, sodium and fluid intake in children with sick cell anaemia. Journal of Blood Disorders Transfer. 2013;**4**(3):1-4. DOI: 10.4172/2155-9864.1000143

[57] Wiebe A, Longbottom J, Gleave K, Shearer FM, Sinka ME, Massey NC, et al. Geographical distributions of African malaria vector sibling species and evidence for insecticide resistance. Malaria Journal. 2017;**16**(1):85

[58] Makani J, Komba AN, Cox SE, Oruo J, Mwamtemi K, Kitundu J, et al. Malaria in patients with sickle

cell anemia: Burden, risk factors, and outcome at the outpatient clinic and during hospitalization. Blood. 2010;**115**:215-220

[59] McAuley CF, Webb C, Makani J, Macharia A, Uyoga S, Opi DH, et al. High mortality from *Plasmodium falciparum* malaria in children living with sickle cell anemia on the coast of Kenya. Blood. 2010;**116**:1663-1668

[60] Frimpong A, Thiam LG, Arko-Boham B, Owusu EDA, Adjei GO. Safety and effectiveness of antimalarial therapy in sickle cell disease: A systematic review and network meta-analysis. BMC Infectious Diseases. 2018;**18**(1):650

[61] Oniyangi O, Omari AA. Malaria chemoprophylaxis in sickle cell disease. Cochrane Database System Review. 2006;**2006**(4):CD003489

[62] Yallop D, Duncan ER, Norris E, Fuller GW, Thomas N, et al. The associations between air quality and the number of hospital admissions for acute pain and sickle-cell disease in an urban environment. British Journal of Haematology. 2007;**136**:844-848

[63] Mekontso Dessap A, Contou D, Dandine-Roulland C, Hemery F, Habibi A, et al. Environmental influences on daily emergency admissions in sickle-cell disease patients. Medicine (Baltimore). 2014;**93**:e280

[64] William BM, Corazza GR. Hyposplenism: A comprehensive review. Part I: Basic concepts and causes. Hema. 2007;**12**(1):1-13

[65] Salawu L, Orimolade EA, Durosinmi MA. Immuno-haematological characteristics of Nigerian sickle cell disease patients in asymptomatic steady state. European Journal of General Medicine. 2009;**6**:170-174

[66] Mousa SA, Al Momen A, Al Sayegh F, Al Jaouni S, Nasrullah Z, Al Saeed H, et al. Management of painful vaso-occlusive crisis of sickle-cell anemia: Consensus opinion. Clinical and Applied Thrombosis/Hemostasis. 2010;**16**(4):365-376

[67] Dieye TN, Ndiaye O, Ndiaye AB, Thiam D, Fall-Seck K, Diop S, et al. Complement and serum immunoglobulins in homozygous and heterozygous sickle cell anemia in Senegal. Dakar Médical. 1999;**44**(2):175-179

[68] Ahmed SG. The role of infection in the pathogenesis of vaso-occlusive crisis in patients with sickle cell disease. MJHID. 2011;**3**(1):e2011028. DOI: 10.4084/MJHID.2011.028

[69] Adzika VA, Glozah FN, Ayim-Aboagye D, Ahorlu CS. Socio-demographic characteristics and psychosocial consequences of sickle cell disease: The case of patients in a public hospital in Ghana. Journal of Health, Population, and Nutrition. 2017;**36**(1):4. DOI: 10.1186/s41043-017-0081-5

[70] Houston-Yu P, Rana SR, Beyer B, et al. Frequent and prolonged hospitalizations: A risk factor for early mortality in sickle cell disease patients. American Journal of Hematology. 2003;**72**(3):201-203

[71] Myrvik MP, Burks LM, Hoffman RG, Dasgupta M, Panepinto JA. Mental health disorders influence admission rates for pain in children with sickle cell disease. Pediatric Blood & Cancer. 2013;**60**(7):1211-1214. DOI: 10.1002/pbc.24394

[72] Myrvik MP, Campbell AD, Davis MM, Butcher JL. Impact of psychiatric diagnoses on hospital length of stay in children with sickle cell anemia. Pediatric Blood & Cancer. 2012;**58**(2):239-243. DOI: 10.1002/pbc.23117

[73] Onyeaka HK, Queeneth U, Rashid W, Ahmad N, Rajan SK, Jaladi PR, et al. Impact of depression in sickle cell disease hospitalization-related outcomes: An Analysis of the National Inpatient Sample (NIS). Medicina (Kaunas, Lithuania). 2019;**55**(7):385. DOI: 10.3390/medicina55070385

[74] Jerrell JM, Tripathi A, McIntyre RS. Prevalence and treatment of depression in children and adolescents with sickle cell disease: A retrospective cohort study. ers. 2011;**13**(2)

[75] Al Zahrani OS, Mukhtar O, Al Subaie M, Al Howiti WE. Systematic psychiatric assessment of patients with sickle cell disease. Saudi Medical Journal. 2019;**40**(1):59-65

[76] Edwards CL, Green M, Wellington CC, Muhammad M, Wood M, Feliu M, et al. Depression, suicidal ideation, and attempts in black patients with sickle cell disease. Journal of the National Medical Association. 2009;**101**: 1090-1095

[77] Al-Marzouki AF, Alrefaie NI, Aljohani NA, Alandanusi RA, Alghamdi AA, Radhwi OO. The prevalence of depression and anxiety among sickle cell disease patients in King Abdulaziz University Hospital. Cureus. 2021;**13**(9):e18374. DOI: 10.7759/cureus.18374

[78] Alhomoud MA, Gosadi IM, Wahbi HA. Depression among sickle cell anemia patients in the Eastern Province of Saudi Arabia. Saudi Journal of Medical Science. 2018;**6**(1):8-12

[79] Ademola Samson Adewoyin. Management of sickle cell disease: A review for physician education in Nigeria (Sub-Saharan Africa). Anaemia. 2015;**2015**:791498. DOI: 10.1155/2015/791498

[80] Jonassaint CR, Kang C, Prussien KV, Yarboi J, Sanger MS, Wilson JD, et al. Feasibility of implementing mobile technology-delivered mental health treatment in routine adult sickle cell disease care. Translational Behavioral Medicine. 2020;**10**(1):58-67

[81] Carroll PC, Haywood C Jr, Hoot MR, Lanzkron SA. preliminary study of psychiatric, familial, and medical characteristics of high-utilizing sickle cell disease patients. The Clinical Journal of Pain. 2013;**29**(4):317-323

[82] Anie KA, Grocott H, White L, et al. Patient self-assessment of hospital pain, mood and health-related quality of life in adults with sickle cell disease. BMJ Open. 2012;**2**:e001274. DOI: 10.1136/bmjopen-2012-001274